Stefanie B. Waller
Renata O. de Faria
Marlete B. Cleff

Medicinal Plants in Sporotrichosis

Stefanie B. Waller
Renata O. de Faria
Marlete B. Cleff

Medicinal Plants in Sporotrichosis

Main botanical families of pharmaceutical interest

ScienciaScripts

Cover image: www.ingimage.com

This book is a translation from the original published under ISBN 978-3-330-77132-1.

Publisher:
Sciencia Scripts
is a trademark of
Dodo Books Indian Ocean Ltd. and OmniScriptum S.R.L publishing group

120 High Road, East Finchley, London, N2 9ED, United Kingdom
Str. Armeneasca 28/1, office 1, Chisinau MD-2012, Republic of Moldova, Europe
Managing Directors: Ieva Konstantinova, Victoria Ursu
info@omniscriptum.com

Printed at: see last page
ISBN: 978-620-8-63600-5

index

INTRODUCTION

Fungal diseases are increasingly important in today's world, affecting humans and animals, especially pediatric and geriatric patients and those with immune deficiencies. Several mycoses are important in human and veterinary medicine, especially those with zoonotic potential, due to their great relevance to public health. Among these infectious diseases, sporotrichosis has been a cause of concern for public health professionals, with increasing cases in humans and animals, especially cats, in recent years.

Sporotrichosis is a subcutaneous infection caused by thermo-dimorphic fungi of the *Sporothrix schenckii* complex and has been recognized as an emerging mycosis with worldwide distribution and a tendency towards exponential growth in the number of cases in humans and animals. In recent years, the disease has been endemic in Central and South American countries such as Mexico, Ecuador, Nicaragua, Venezuela, Colombia, Uruguay, Peru and Brazil.

Sporadic cases have been described mainly in humans in European countries such as Ireland, France, Italy, Bulgaria, among others. On the African continent, the countries of Egypt, Nigeria and South Africa have also reported the occurrence of the disease, as well as on the Asian continent, where Iran, Nepal, Thailand, Laos, Malaysia, China, South Korea and, above all, India and Japan, have warned about the high incidence of this mycosis. In Oceania, human sporotrichosis has been reported through classical transmission.

In Brazil, the main reports occur in the Southeast and South regions, especially in the states of Rio de Janeiro and Rio Grande do Sul, where transmission by scratching and/or biting healthy and sick cats has been highlighted as the main form of contagion.

The disease presents clinically, in animals and humans, with lesions subcutaneous nodular, ulcerative and crusted in different regions of the body, and can involve the lymphatic system and spread to internal organs. Thus, the clinical presentations of the disease are characterized by fixed cutaneous, disseminated cutaneous, lymphocutaneous and systemic and\or disseminated forms. Different antifungal therapies are recommended for animals, as the different clinical presentations of the disease require different therapeutic protocols.

Historically, sodium and potassium iodides were the first antifungals used in the treatment of human and animal sporotrichosis in the 20th century, and over the years they were replaced by new antifungals created by the pharmaceutical industry. The advent of azole drugs, such as ketoconazole and especially itraconazole, marked the era of successful antifungal therapy with fewer adverse effects and clinical cures for animals.

Other therapeutic classes have been studied and used, such as amphotericin B and terbinafine, but their use has been more frequent in the treatment of human sporotrichosis than in the disease in dogs and cats.

Prolonged antifungal therapy is recognized for a minimum period of three to five months, and should be extended for at least another month once the clinical signs have subsided. However, this therapeutic management has not been respected by those responsible for medicating animals with the disease.

Veterinary therapy is not an isolated practice and is closely related to the commitment and responsibility of the guardian during the treatment of the animals. The difficulties encountered in therapeutic management include the high cost of the drug and prolonged treatment time, and therapeutic failures are observed due to inadequate administration and pharmacological quality, as well as animal receptivity and the ability of the guardian. Thus, the commitment of the guardian is essential for the therapeutic success of sporotrichosis in animals.

In the presence of these difficulties, there is a risk of the fungal agent becoming resistant to drugs, which has been observed in fungi of the *Sporothrix schenckii* complex. This scenario reinforces the need to research alternatives for the treatment of sporotrichosis using chemical compounds with antifungal activity, especially medicinal plants.

Although allopathic therapies are common practice, new molecules have been researched nationally and internationally, based on plant extracts, with the aim of finding potential alternative products with antifungal activities against the agents of sporotrichosis. Especially in countries with a rich biodiversity, such as Brazil, various botanical species have been used in experimental trials and have shown excellent antifungal activities. The use of flora as therapeutic products has been promising in terms of sustainability and affordability.

Extracts from plants belonging to different botanical families have been studied for their potential activity against fungi of the complex

Sporothrix schenckii, with emphasis on the families Lamiaceae, Combretaceae, Asteraceae, Myrtaceae, Fabaceae, Anacardiaceae, Agavaceae, Polygalaceae, Poaceae and others, constituting at least 81 botanical species already investigated worldwide.

This book provides up-to-date information on the future prospects for the treatment of sporotrichosis in canines and felines, and focuses on the prospecting of bioactive medicinal plants for this purpose. In addition, it covers epidemiological, clinical and therapeutic information on sporotrichosis and its importance in public health, describing the current scenario of the disease in Brazil and alerting health professionals to the problem of antifungal resistance observed in the *Sporothrix schenckii* complex.

CHAPTER 1

Sporotrichosis and the *Sporothrix schenckii* Complex

Sporotrichosis is a subcutaneous mycosis caused by pathogenic fungi belonging to the *Sporothrix schenckii* complex. Although the species *Sporothrix schenckii* has been considered the sole etiologic agent of the disease for many years, recent research related to the phylogenetic analysis of clinical isolates from humans and animals has revealed that the disease is caused by a complex of pathogenic species of the genus *Sporothrix*. Around 50 species are known as non-pathogenic environmental fungi and are geophilic agents present in plants, wood and soil. Of these species, some have pathogenic potential for humans and animals, mainly the species *Sporothrix brasiliensis*, *S. schenckii* sensu stricto, *S. globosa*, *S. luriei*, *S. mexicana* and *S. chilensis*.

Sporotrichosis is recognized worldwide and several geographical areas have declared it an emerging public health problem. Although the disease is frequent in tropical and subtropical regions, increasing reports have been described in countries in Africa, Asia and Central and South America, especially Brazil, Mexico, Colombia, Peru and Uruguay, as well as Japan, South Africa and India. Although less frequent in Europe, sporotrichosis was a common disease in France in the early 1900s, and has now been described in sporadic cases in Italy, Portugal, Spain and Turkey.

In animals, sporotrichosis has been described in dogs and cats in the United States, Canada, Italy, India, Japan and Malaysia, with Brazil being considered one of the South American countries with a high prevalence of the disease in small animals.

The first case of human sporotrichosis in Brazil was reported in a patient from São Paulo in 1902. In veterinary medicine, the first record of feline sporotrichosis was in 1954, in an animal from the state of Minas Gerais, in the city of Cambuquira. Canine sporotrichosis was described for the first time in

1957, in a dog from Santa Catarina.

Currently, sporadic cases occur in the states of Mato Grosso, Espirito Santo, Rio Grande do Norte, Minas Gerais, São Paulo, Paranà and Santa Catarina. However, the states of Rio de Janeiro and Rio Grande do Sul have frequent cases in humans and animals, and are considered endemic regions for the disease.

Of the pathogenic species of the *Sporothrix schenckii* complex, phylogenetic studies have identified the *S. globosa* species as prevalent in clinical cases of the disease in Spain, Italy, Japan, India and the United States. *Sporothrix globosa* has also been isolated from environmental samples of soil, wheat and sugar cane in China. In Germany, fungal isolation from wheat fields has isolated *S. inflata*, while *S. mexicana* has been isolated from soil, rose bushes and carnation leaves in Mexico.

Clinical cases of sporotrichosis by *S. schenckii* have been identified in sick humans in the United States, Peru, Argentina, Venezuela, Colombia, Bolivia and South Africa, as well as by *S. schenckii* var. *luriei* in cases of human sporotrichosis in South Africa.

The *S. brasiliensis* species is currently recognized as exclusive to Brazil, with no record of its fungal isolation in any other geographical region of the world. This pathogenic species has been reported with a high prevalence in cases of feline sporotrichosis outbreaks, and its high virulence has worried health professionals about controlling the disease in animals and humans. Currently, *S. brasiliensis* is considered the most pathogenic species among the agents of the *Sporothrix schenckii* complex.

1.1. Epidemiological aspects

1.1.1. Disease Transmission

Sporotrichosis is transmitted by inoculating the fungus into the skin tissue through trauma. The fungal microorganism can present itself in both dimorphic phases, triggering the disease in a chronic or subacute form depending on the host's immune status. Although occasional and sporadic, infection by inhalation of fungal conidia can occur, developing pulmonary sporotrichosis.

1.1.1.1. Environmental Contact: "The Rose Disease"

As a saprobic and geophilic fungus, *Sporothrix* spp. are naturally present in environmental sources such as wood splinters, plant thorns and stems, soil rich in organic matter, etc., and their morphological phase is filamentous. Thus, direct physical contact with traumatic involvement of the skin by sharp materials, containing the conidia, corresponds to the most common transmission of the disease in the world. In the past, the disease was occupational in people working in agriculture, gardening and logging, and was recognized as "rose disease" due to the frequency of the disease in patients with traumatic contact with the thorns of these plants.

In this type of infection, the microorganism inoculated by the filamentous phase begins the process of disappearing the fungal hyphae between 24 and 48 hours after traumatic inoculation. In approximately 13 days, the agent completes the process of morphological transition to the leveduriform phase in order to survive in the host organism. The incubation period for filamentous inoculation of the agent is longer and ranges from one week to one month.

1.1.1.2. Animal Contact: Zoonotic Disease

In turn, *Sporothrix* spp. can also be transmitted when it is in the leveduriform stage, a parasitic stage that is transmitted through the scratching and biting of infected felines. When an animal or human is infected by the agent at this stage, the microorganism is already in adaptable conditions for parasitism and therefore starts cell multiplication immediately, as it lacks morphological transition. This form of transmission is the most common in Brazil's endemic regions, such as Rio de Janeiro and Rio Grande do Sul, which occurs through zoonotic involvement via scratches and/or bites from infected felines. Cats account for the largest number of reported cases and are considered the main transmitters of the disease to other animals and to humans (Figure 1).

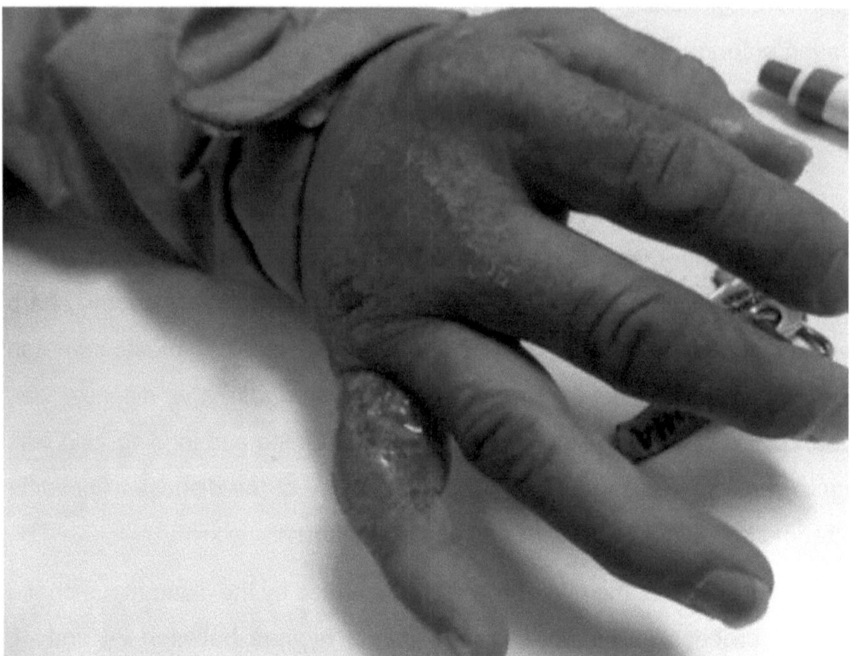

Figure 1 - Ulcerative and suppurative lesion on the third phalanx of the fifth finger of the right hand of a male patient, resident in the city of Pelotas, Rio Grande do Sul (Brazil) due to zoonotic transmission by a feline (Veterinary Mycology Diagnostic and Research Center, Federal University of Pelotas, RS, Brazil).

1.1.2. Risk Species

Due to the geophilic characteristics of the fungus and the type of transmission, any animal species is subject to traumatic involvement of the skin by contaminated sharps and is at risk of developing sporotrichosis. In addition to humans, dogs and cats have a high frequency of the disease in Brazil. Other animals have been reported with sporotrichosis, such as armadillos, dolphins, horses, cattle, camels, rabbits, foxes, pigs, rats, mice and chimpanzees.

In humans, the disease had a high incidence in farmers, gardeners, logging workers, among others, who represent the risk group for the disease, due to intimate contact with contaminated plant material without protection. However, sporadic cases or small outbreaks currently occur among rural workers in Brazil. In endemic areas, the main form of transmission has been related to zoonotic involvement through scratches and/or bites from infected cats. The main risk group is therefore cat owners and veterinary surgeons, especially those who have direct contact with sick animals.

1.1.3. The Role of Domestic Cats

Currently, domestic cats play an important role in the spread of sporotrichosis, due to the possibility of transmitting the disease through scratches and/or bites. Through the routine habit of digging in the ground and sharpening their nails on tree trunks, which favor contact with *Sporothrix* spp. present in the environment, cats can carry the agent to the oral cavity by body hygiene through licking.

Transmission to other animals and to humans is facilitated in this species, since the projection of its nails and teeth makes it easier to cause skin trauma during fights and games.

In addition, the great zoonotic potential of felines is also due to the fact that cats with mycosis contain numerous *Sporothrix* spp. cells in the yeast stage in their lesions, which is rarely seen in humans and canines. In addition, there is currently a greater proximity of felines to humans as pets in Brazil, which favors physical contact and the spread of the disease. Therefore, the feline species has been associated with the highest number of reported cases of sporotrichosis and is considered the main inter- and intra-species transmitter of the disease.

The cats most at risk of being involved with the disease, and consequently of transmitting it, are those that are peridomiciled or free-living, especially unspayed males of reproductive age, due to the fact that they are often involved in territorial and reproductive disputes over females.

1.2 Clinical signs

The host's immunity can contribute to the lesion remaining in the inoculated spot until it involutes spontaneously, leaving an "immunological scar", which is seen in humans through positive intradermal tests for the sporotrichin protein.

However, the fungus's pathogenicity factors, such as thermotolerance, the presence of melanin, extracellular enzymes and cell wall constituents, make it difficult for the immune system to fight the agent. These factors facilitate the onset of fungal infection and the consequent development of clinical lesions, which take between 2 and 24 months to develop.

The clinical presentations of sporotrichosis commonly occur in the cutaneous and cutaneous-lymphatic forms, with the systemic form being rare, in which patients with immunosuppression present involvement of organs such as the liver and spleen, through lymphatic and hematogenous dissemination. The host's skin lesions appear anywhere on the body, usually from the site of traumatic inoculation.

Thus, the clinical signs manifest themselves in humans and animals through nodules which tend to ulcerate over time, releasing draining exudate and even purulent secretion, and which can involve the lymphatic system. The main regions affected in animals are the head, face, trunk, extremities and tail.

Although occasional and sporadic, infection by inhalation of fungal conidia can occur, developing pulmonary sporotrichosis. The signs are manifested by dyspnea, nasal discharge and sneezing, especially in cases of traumatic fungal inoculation in the nasal plane, associated with alveolar edema. In severe cases, the lesions can develop into necrosis with exposure of muscles and even bones, especially in cats.

In canines, cutaneous sporotrichosis with multiple firm nodules, alopecic areas and ulcerated lesions that are not pruritic and not painful are common. The most affected regions are the head, ears and trunk, with the nasal plane being the most susceptible area (Figure 2). This is due to the fact that, in a fight or game between dogs and cats, the canine nasal area is highly susceptible to scratches from felines that can carry and transmit the agent.

Nodular lesions tend to be firm, ulcerated and with the presence of purulent exudate and crusts, and generally without pruritus. On the other hand, signs of dermatitis with itching and weight loss have also been reported in some dogs with sporotrichosis.

The cutaneous-lymphatic form can occur, with the manifestation of nodules on the limbs, for example, and consequent ascending infection via the lymphatic route. In some more serious cases, the disease can spread to vital organs, seriously compromising the health of the animals, but this widespread manifestation is considered rare.

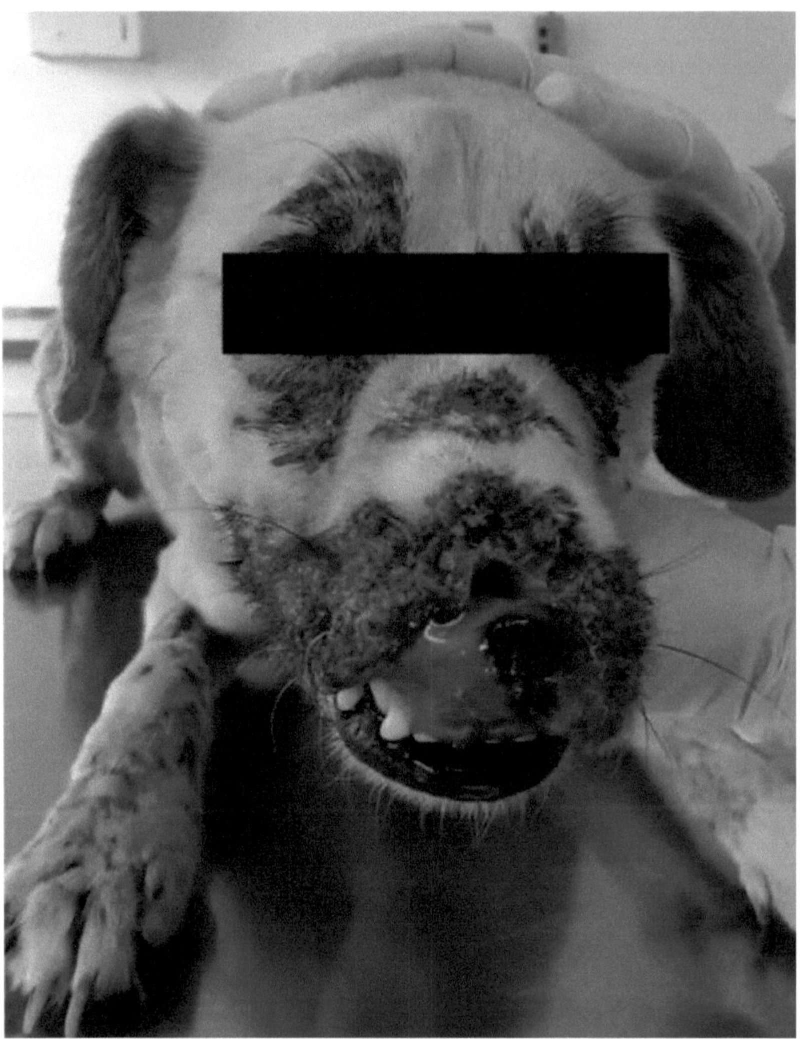

Figura 2. Sporotrichosis in the nasal planum of a female canine resident in the city of Cerrito, Rio Grande do Sul (Brazil), with destruction of the region and presence of secondary infection (GUTERRES et al., 2014), diagnosed by the Center for Diagnosis and Research in Veterinary Mycology (Federal University of Pelotas, RS, Brazil).

In cats, sporotrichosis has different clinical manifestations, which can be single or multiple skin lesions all over the body. The cutaneous and lymphocutaneous form are the most common presentations, and the main signs include papulonodular lesions, which ulcerate and release serous exudate. The lesions often become purulent and even bloody, and can develop into thick crusts.

In some cases, adjacent lymphatic vessels are compromised. Although lesions can occur in any area of the body, the most common in cats are the head (Figure 3), face, trunk, extremities and tail.

Respiratory signs include dyspnea, nasal discharge and sneezing, especially in cases of traumatic fungal inoculation of the nasal planum, associated with alveolar edema. Thus, deformation of the nasal plan with stenosis and even exposure of the nasal orifices can also occur. Other signs are observed, such as apathy, depression, hyperthermia and dehydration.

Cats with sporotrichosis have a high number of *Sporothrix* spp. yeast cells in their clinical lesions. This is an inherent characteristic of this animal species and, for this reason, areas of necrosis are frequently observed. In addition, severe cases of the disease can lead to the spread of the fungal agent to other parts of the body, including vital organs such as the lungs, liver, gastrointestinal tract, central nervous system, joints, bones, kidneys and testicles.

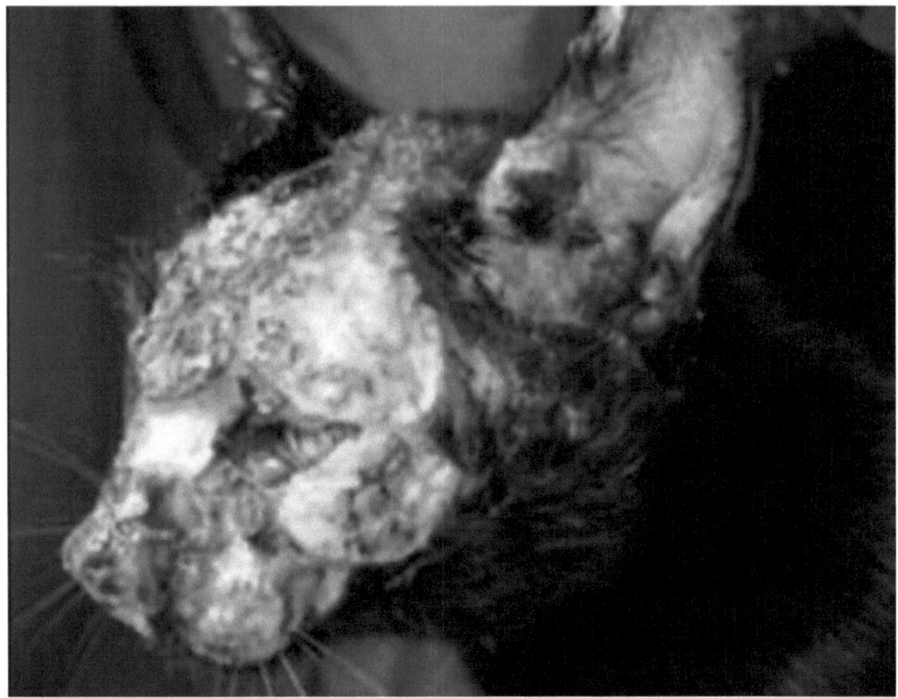

Figura 3. Cutaneous sporotrichosis located on the face of a domestic feline living in the city of Pelotas, Rio Grande do Sul (Brazil), with extensive ulcerative and crusted lesions with the presence of bloody exudate (Center for Diagnosis and Research in Veterinary Mycology, Federal University of Pelotas, RS, Brazil).

1.3. Disease Diagnosis

In order to diagnose sporotrichosis with certainty, the animal's history, anamnesis, clinical signs and isolation of *Sporothrix* spp. in culture media from clinical material collected from the suspect animal must be associated.

1.3.1. Clinical Sample Collection and Processing

For clinical collection, sterile *swabs* should be pressed into the skin lesions, which should then be cleaned by spraying them with physiological solution or sterile solution. In the case of nodular lesions, prior antiseptic cleaning with 70°GL alcohol should be carried out, and clinical samples collected by means of skin biopsy or fine needle aspiration. In these cases, the samples should be sent immediately for mycological analysis within 24 hours, or kept refrigerated.

For histopathological analysis, the sample should be kept in 10% formalin for fixation. Samples of crusts or exudates can be collected by scraping the skin with a sterile scalpel, and blood samples collected without anticoagulants can be used.

By directly examining clinical samples, such as exudates, tissues or aspirates from lesions, it is possible to visualize the yeast-like structures of *Sporothrix* spp. using Gram staining. This visualization is common in samples from sick cats, as this species has a large number of fungal structures in clinical lesions. However, direct visualization is rare in other animal species, such as humans and dogs.

1.3.2. Fungic cultivation

Mycological cultivation is an essential analysis for confirming the disease. Various culture media can be used, such as Sabouraud-dextrose agar, Potato-dextrose agar, Brain and Heart Infusion agar, with or without antimicrobials, and kept at 25°C and 37°C for a period of 5 to 15 days, to confirm the characteristic fungal dimorphism and the macro and micromorphological evaluation of the colonies. After fungal growth, the macromorphological analysis is initially observed through the characteristics of the colonies, followed by microscopic analysis.

In the filamentous phase grown between 25° and 27°C, the colonies are wrinkled with irradiated edges resembling a star-shaped appearance, adherent to the culture medium and may present a resistant film formed by an interlacing of hyphae. The color varies from cream to gray, and can darken to a dark gray to black color. This pigmentation is associated with the production of melanin by the fungus, which is considered to be one of the main virulence factors of the *Sporothrix schenckii* complex. In direct microscopy of filamentous colonies, the fungal material should be placed between a slide and a coverslip containing a drop of lactophenol blue and evaluated at 400x magnification, to observe numerous hyaline and septate hyphae with conidiophores containing abundant conidia at their "daisy"-shaped ends (Figure 4).

In the yeast phase, which grows between 35° and 37°C, the colonies have a creamy appearance and vary in color from light to beige. Microscopic examination of the colonies in this phase is carried out using the Gram technique, at 1000x magnification with immersion oil, where round, oval or cigar-shaped cells are observed, which can be found free or phagocytized, containing a clear halo (Figure 5).

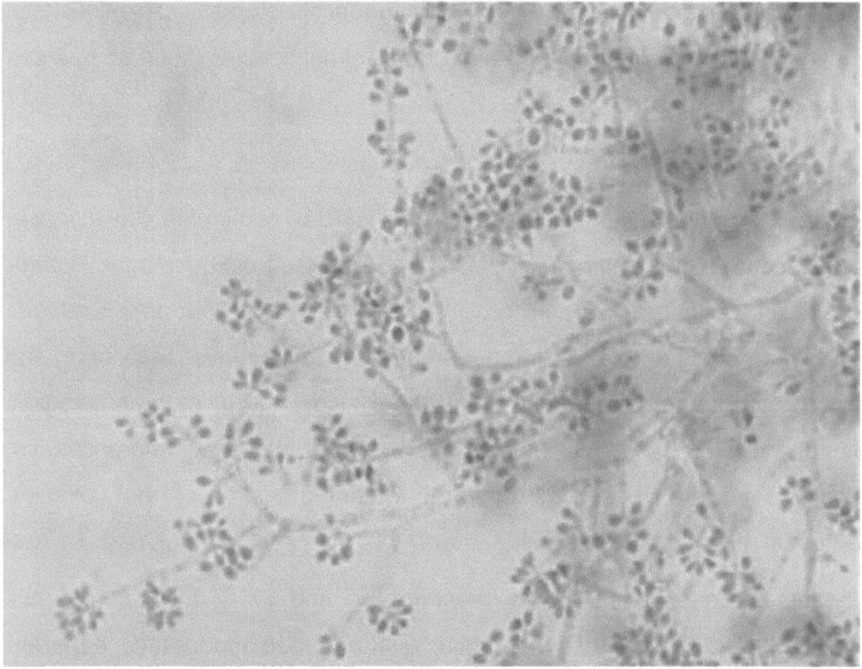

Figura 4. Microscopic appearance of *Sporothrix* spp. in the filamentous phase, with the presence of numerous hyphae containing dispersed conidia in an arrangement similar to a "daisy flower". Staining with Lactophenol Cotton Blue. 400x magnification (Veterinary Mycology Diagnostic and Research Center, Federal University of Pelotas, RS, Brazil).

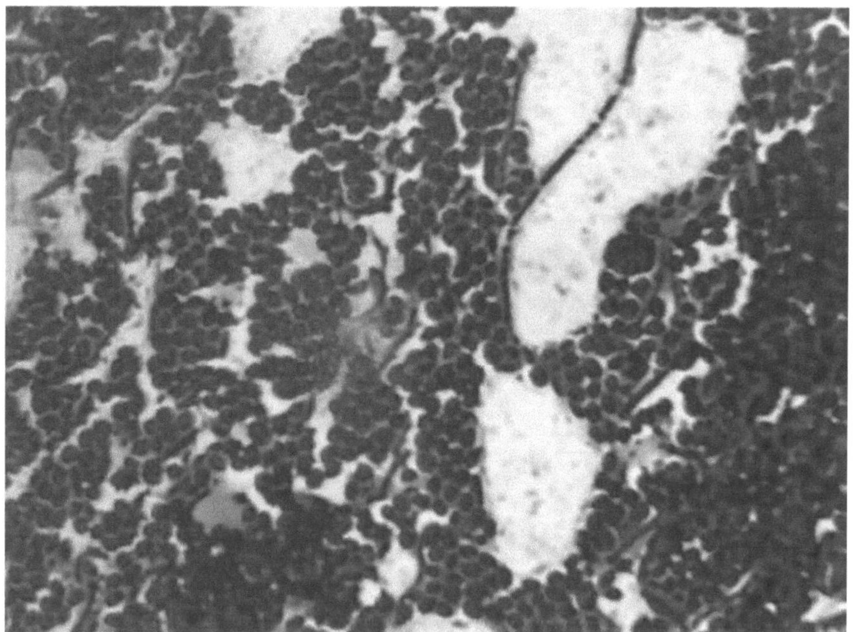

Figura 5. Microscopic appearance of *Sporothrix* spp. in the yeast-like phase, where oval to elongated "cigar-shaped" cells can be seen; there is also a morphological transition from some yeast-like cells to filamentous cells, starting with the presence of hyphae. Gram stain. 400x magnification (Veterinary Mycology Diagnostic and Research Center, Federal University of Pelotas, RS, Brazil).

1.3.3. Histopathological analysis

In the histopathological examination, tissues fixed in 10% formalin can be subjected to the histochemical staining techniques of Hematoxylin-Eosin (H.E.), Periodoic Acid Schiff (PAS) and Gomori's Arsenic Methenamine.), Periodic Acid Schiff (PAS) and Gomori's Methenamine Arsenic staining techniques, which make it possible to see the yeast cells of the *Sporothrix* spp. which, in general, are intracellular, with an oval to elongated, cigar-like appearance, and may have single or multiple sprouts.

Visualization of fungal structures is easier in samples from cats, but more difficult in humans and dogs, even in the presence of active lesions and with isolation of the agent. In H.E. staining, cells from the inflammatory infiltrate, such as macrophages, giant cells, neutrophils and lymphocytes are commonly observed. In samples from dogs and cats with sporotrichosis, the findings are characterized by acanthotic and ulcerated epidermis, with the presence of crusts and exudation.

Findings suggestive of sporotrichosis are the asteroid corpuscles, also known as the Splendore-Hoeppli phenomenon, which are the parasitic forms of *Sporothrix* spp. coated with immunoglobulins, although this is not a pathognomonic finding of the disease.

In addition, the visualization of granulomas caused by *Sporothrix* spp. are usually presented with a necrotic suppurative center surrounded by epithelioid granulomatous inflammation, which show a high number of giant, multinucleated cells and a lymphoplasmocytic halo with granulation tissue and fibrosis.

1.3.4. Inoculation in Experimental Animals

Inoculation in laboratory animals can be carried out using suspensions of fungal cells or pathological material via the subcutaneous, intraperitoneal or even intratesticular routes. This procedure makes it possible to observe the pathogenicity of the agent in animals by observing the specific clinical signs of the disease.

Subsequently, the animal is euthanized and submitted to necropsy, where the clinical material is collected and submitted to retroisolation of *Sporothrix* spp. in the laboratory. It should be noted that the use of experimental infection in laboratory animals has not been used in routine diagnostics in recent years, but is more used for scientific research purposes, where the use of animals must follow the criteria established by committees and bodies responsible for animal welfare.

1.3.5. Sporotrichin skin test

The sporotrichin protein can be used in patients as an intradermal reaction test

. It is most commonly used in human patients, especially for epidemiological surveys of the disease. Once the substance has been applied and a positive skin reaction has been observed, this test indicates the existence of previous contact between the host and the fungal agent, however, cross-reactions with other diseases can occur, resulting in false positives.

If there is no skin reaction, this test allows us to conclude that the disease is absent in the host. In dogs, the sporotrichin test can be used to differentiate sporotrichosis from leishmaniasis.

1.3.6. Serology

Through the blood sample collected without anticoagulant, the serological material is separated from the clot and can be used in serological techniques for the diagnosis of sporotrichosis, such as complement fixation, immunodiffusion, agglutination on latex particles, ELISA and indirect immunofluorescence. These tests are frequently used in suspected cases of human sporotrichosis and, of the techniques mentioned, latex agglutination is the most suitable, as it is a highly specific and sensitive test for the agent.

1.3.7. Differential Diagnosis

The clinical signs of sporotrichosis are similar to those of other diseases in dogs and cats, which should be taken into account when assessing the diagnosis. These include leishmaniasis, cryptococcosis, mycobacteriosis, pyoderma and neoplasms such as squamous cell carcinoma, which are frequently seen in cats. Complementary tests are essential for a correct clinical diagnosis.

CHAPTER 2

Conventional Therapy in Veterinary Medicine

Various antifungal drugs are used to treat the disease in humans and animals, such as potassium iodide, itraconazole, ketoconazole, amphotericin B and terbinafine. Other therapies can be used in association with antifungal treatment, such as the use of surgical techniques and other non-drug modalities.

Obtaining a clinical cure depends on factors related to the therapy, such as cost, route of administration, pharmacological safety and sensitivity of the agent. In addition, severe clinical and systemic cases of infection require more aggressive treatment, even if the risks of drug toxicity are higher.

On average, treatment time varies from 3 to 6 months and should be maintained for 4 to 6 weeks after the clinical signs have subsided, making correct therapeutic management crucial.

Unfortunately, the indiscriminate and inadequate use of antifungal drugs has favored the emergence of resistant strains *of Sporothrix* spp. making it difficult to control in many clinical cases, as well as costly to obtain a clinical cure.

2.1. Sodium and Potassium Iodides

At the beginning of the 20th century, iodides were the first drugs to be used to treat localized sporotrichosis in humans, and years later they were used in animals. They are inexpensive and have been effective in cases refractory to itraconazole. In cats, the recommended dose is 10 to 20 mg/kg every 12 or 24 hours, orally, while in dogs, a 20% saturated solution of sodium or potassium iodide is recommended at a dose of 40 mg/kg every 8 hours, extending therapy for both species for a further 30 days once the lesions have cleared up. In the form of oral capsules, potassium iodide is highly effective when used in cats at doses of 2.5 to 20 mg/kg/day, and is successfully recommended in cases refractory to the use of itraconazole alone.

Although the mechanism of action has not yet been elucidated, it is believed that iodides are converted into iodine by the enzyme *myeloperoxidase*, thus having a fungicidal action. Furthermore, the antifungal activity has been related to phagocytosis, by inhibiting the formation of granulomas through immunological and non-immunological mechanisms, exposing the *Sporothrix* spp. to the host's defense cells and to the antifungals circulating in the body.

It is highly recommended to monitor liver enzyme levels, due to the hepatotoxic potential of iodides, as well as to observe the possible side effects of iodism, such as anorexia, lethargy, fever, vomiting, diarrhea, hyperexcitability and cardiomyopathy, especially in cats.

Dogs may show epiphora, a runny nose and a dry coat and, in these conditions, the drug should be suspended for around 7 days and the dose gradually increased. Potassium iodide is also contraindicated during pregnancy.

2.2. Azolic drugs

With good antifungal activity because they bind to fungal cytochrome P450, azoles promote activity against *Sporothrix* spp. by inhibiting demethylation of the ergosterol precursor, lanosterol, and consequently inhibiting ergosterol synthesis, altering fungal membrane permeability.

2.2.1. Ketoconazole

At the end of the 1970s, ketoconazole emerged as a promising drug and was used orally in feline therapy at doses of 10 to 50 mg/kg/day and in canines at doses of 5 to 15 mg/kg every 12 hours. Studies have shown that ketoconazole has good *in vitro* activity against the species *S. brasiliensis, S. schenckii* and *S. globosa*, which showed greater sensitivity, but it did not work well against *S. albicans* and *S. mexicana*.

Ketoconazole is well absorbed when in contact with acidic pH, and its administration during meals is indicated. Pharmacological metabolization occurs at the hepatic level, allowing the use of this drug in patients with renal insufficiency, however, monitoring serum levels of hepatic transaminases is essential during treatment.

However, ketoconazole has a slow response compared to other antifungals, and is not recommended in cases of disseminated sporotrichosis. In addition, adverse effects can occur, such as vomiting, nausea, diarrhea, inappetence and, above all, hepatotoxic effects, and its use is prohibited in pregnancy due to its teratogenic and embryotoxic potential.

2.2.2. Itraconazole

Introduced in the 1990s, itraconazole represented a new generation of antifungals for systemic use on the pharmaceutical market, because although it has the same mechanism of action as ketoconazole, it has a high affinity for fungal cytochrome P450, with an action 5 to 100 times more potent and selective in the fungal cell. Because it is a triazole derivative, itraconazole has three nitrogen atoms in the azole ring in its chemical structure, which gives it little binding to the cytochrome P450 of mammalian cells, making it less toxic than other antifungals. For this reason, itraconazole has been recognized as the drug of choice in feline and canine sporotrichosis.

The success of itraconazole treatment in cats and dogs is achieved at a dose of 10 to 40 mg/kg/day, orally, for at least three months, and should be extended for at least 30 days after the cure. The average time to clinical cure is between 3 and 6 months for felines at the above dose and around 6 to 11 months for canines, with no adverse effects.

Used orally, itraconazole is highly lipophilic, with excellent absorption after food administration, with a peak plasma concentration of around 3 hours and a plasma half-life of 8 to 12 hours. Itraconazole is often used in the commercial form of oral capsules, although the concentrations available for veterinary use are limited. As they do not meet the concentrations recommended for animal patients, the use of manipulated medicines has been frequent and the use of manipulated itraconazole has demonstrated fungistatic activity *in vitro* against

Sporothrix spp.

Of the species of the *Sporothrix schenckii* complex, *S. schenckii, S. globosa, S. albicans and S. mexicana* from human clinical cases have been sensitive to itraconazole, especially *S. brasiliensis*. Compared to other drugs, itraconazole has shown a better response than voriconazole and terbinafine.

Although the adverse effects of itraconazole in cats are rare, gastrointestinal effects, such as nausea, vomiting and abdominal discomfort, and hepatotoxic effects may occur, and the drug should be temporarily suspended until liver enzymes normalize. Itraconazole has a potent embryotoxic and teratogenic effect and should not be used during pregnancy. In addition, its use requires a prolonged period of treatment, ranging from three to six months, and is expensive.

2.2.3. Fluconazole

Fluconazole is also an azole antifungal and is recommended at a dose of 10 mg/kg, every 24 hours, orally. Its use in cats has promoted the remission of skin lesions and respiratory signs in 3 months of treatment, with no adverse effects. However, it is rarely used *in vivo,* and *in vitro* studies have shown its weak or no activity against *S. brasiliensis, S. schenckii, S. globosa, S. mexicana* and *S. albicans*.

2.3. Terbinafine

From the group of allylamines, the antifungal action of terbinafine is due to the selective inhibition of the enzyme *squalene-epoxidase*, which is involved in the synthesis of ergosterol, vital for the formation of the plasma membrane, and, in addition, the accumulation of squalene inside the cell is toxic to the fungal cell.

Terbinafine is recommended for cats with sporotrichosis at a dose of 30 mg/kg/day alone or in combination with itraconazole. When administered orally, it is biotransformed in the liver by the P450 system and rapidly absorbed and taken up by the skin, nail and adipose tissue, while topically, it easily penetrates the skin tissue. As it is highly lipophilic, its antifungal activity remains in adipose tissue for a few weeks after stopping the drug.

The high activity of terbinafine against *S. brasiliensis, S. schenckii, S. globosa, S. mexicana* and *S. albicans* has been demonstrated *in vitro*, even compared to amphotericin B antifungals and traditional and modern azole drugs, such as posaconazole and voriconazole. In *S. globosa* and *S. schenckii* resistant to itraconazole, terbinafine has been a therapeutic option.

In vitro tests have shown that the combination of terbinafine with itraconazole and the combination of terbinafine with ketoconazole showed better antifungal activity compared to the use of these drugs alone, which could be an option for clinical cases refractory to itraconazole. However, its efficacy *in vivo* needs to be better studied, and the high cost of terbinafine is a barrier to its therapeutic use in some countries, which is also observed in veterinary medicine.

2.4. Amphotericin B

Produced by *Streptomyces nodosus*, amphotericin B is a polyene antibiotic because it has several double bonds in its chemical composition and its antifungal activity is due to its ability to bind irreversibly to ergosterol, promoting the release of potassium and magnesium ions, which compromise fungal metabolism.

Amphotericin B is recommended at a dose of 0.15 to 0.5 mg/kg/day, intravenously, every other day, for a total dose of 4 to 12 mg/kg. Few studies have reported the use of amphotericin B in feline sporotrichosis, which is used intravenously and intralesionally, the latter being indicated in clinical cases refractory to itraconazole.

The combined use of intralesional amphotericin B (1 mg/kg) with oral itraconazole (20 mg/kg) has been used successfully in cats with localized cutaneous sporotrichosis refractory to itraconazole. *In in vitro* studies, amphotericin B has shown activity against *S. brasiliensis* and *S. schenckii*, but *S. globosa, S. albicans* and *S. mexicana* were not sensitive to this drug. In addition, a comparative study of cutaneous sporotrichosis in Wistar rats demonstrated the weak action of amphotericin B at a dose of 20 to 30 mg/kg, compared to itraconazole administered at 10 mg/kg, which showed better results.

Although doses higher than 1 mg/kg/day are more effective, their use is limited in dogs and cats, due to the nephrotoxic effects triggered by the drug's greater affinity for cholesterol in the host's cell membrane. Renal toxicity can be observed as an adverse effect, due to a decrease in the glomerular filtration rate, since amphotericin B has a constrictive effect on the afferent arterioles, and its use should be suspended when signs of hypokalemia and hypomagnesemia are observed. Patients receiving amphotericin B should be intensely hydrated in order to reduce the chances of nephrotoxic effects.

liposomal amphotericin B formulations are currently on the market with reduced toxic effects, but at higher prices. With regard to pregnancy, its use is permitted with constant monitoring. In pregnant women, the use of amphotericin B for 12 months promoted cure clinical without adverse effects, however, this drug is reserved for pulmonary and disseminated cases.

2.5. Flucitocin

Also known as 5-fluocytokine, flucitone acts on various enzymes that activate its compound 5-fluoracil into 5-fluoro-2'-deoxyuridine-5'- monophosphate, a substance that inhibits the enzyme *thymidylate synthetase* from synthesizing fungal DNA. Although little used in animal sporotrichosis, its use is recommended at a dose of 125 to 250 mg/kg/day, orally.

However, species of the *Sporothrix schenckii* complex have been weakly sensitive to flucytokine, especially *S. brasiliensis*, *S. mexicana* and *S. albicans.* Side effects include anemia, leukopenia, thrombocytopenia, nausea, vomiting, diarrhea, severe enterocolitis and hepatomegaly, and its use should be discontinued and signs monitored.

2.6. New antifungal drugs

In studies with drugs of the echinocandin class, which inhibit the enzyme *glucan synthetase* involved in the synthesis of β-glucan, an important component in the formation of the fungal cell wall, the results against the *Sporothrix schenckii* complex have not been satisfactory. Caspofungin was weakly active *in vitro* against *S. brasiliensis, S. schenckii, S. globosa* and *S. mexicana*, as was micafungin, whose MIC values were 256 µg⁄ml for the species of the *Sporothrix schenckii* complex, considered extremely high and without activity.

New triazole drugs have been studied in sporotrichosis with promising results *in vitro*, especially posaconazole, which obtained better activity than other drugs, such as amphotericin B and itraconazole, against *S. brasiliensis, S. schenckii, S. globosa* and *S. albicans*, even with MICs lower than or equal to 2 µg√ml against *S. brasiliensis* and *S. schenckii*.

Posaconazole has also been effective in murine models of infection with *S. brasiliensis* and *S. schenckii*, including when this drug is combined with amphotericin B, where its synergistic effect has been effective in experimental disseminated sporotrichosis caused by *S. brasiliensis*, showing promise for the treatment of dogs and cats with the disease. However, posaconazole is not widely available in Brazil and is used with restrictions due to its cost, but it could be a therapeutic option in the future.

Other modern triazoles have been active *in vitro*, although their therapeutic efficiency can be interfered with by the fungal species. In albaconazole and ravuconazole, *S. brasiliensis* has been sensitive at MICs between 0.25 and 4 µgλml and 0.5 and 16 µg⅛ respectively, however, the same drugs have not been effective against *S. schenckii*, *S. globosa, S. mexicana S. albicans*.

The same was observed with voriconazole in a murine model in mice with disseminated sporotrichosis, which were treated orally (40 mg/kg/day), with better therapeutic efficiency observed in animals infected with *S. schenckii* compared to those infected with *S. brasiliensis*, whose drug was weakly active.

On the other hand, studies have shown that voriconazole is weak *in vitro* against species of the *Sporothrix schenckii* complex. When combined with another antifungal drug, voriconazole showed no advantage in drug interaction with terbinafine, having an indifferent or even antagonistic effect, making its use poorly recommended in the treatment of sporotrichosis.

2.7. Other Therapeutic Options

2.7.1. Surgical Procedures

In cases refractory to itraconazole, the combination of an antifungal and a surgical procedure may be an alternative. In a clinical case of feline sporotrichosis refractory to itraconazole, a cat with a lesion located in the scrotum was clinically cured after orchiectomy and excision of the scrotum and antifungal therapy with itraconazole (20 mg/kg/day) for 2 months. This modality could be an option for drug-refractory cases, but it has the disadvantage of limiting the location of the lesion in different anatomical sites, as it is only allowed in places where surgical intervention is possible.

The use of cryosurgery associated with antifungal drugs is also an alternative. The combination of itraconazole (10 mg/kg) with the liquid nitrogen freezing procedure on the skin lesions of cats with sporotrichosis has been successfully studied. Researchers have emphasized the importance of continuing treatment at the same dosage for a further four weeks from the time of complete remission of the lesions, in order to increase the chances of a cure, the average time of which has been 32 weeks.

2.7.2. Use of Immunomodulatory Substance

Another alternative in cases refractory to itraconazole is the use of immunomodulatory substances such as (1-3)-β-glucan. This polysaccharide is a compound extracted from the inner cell wall of the fungus *Saccharomyces cerevisiae* and has immunostimulant activity in the mammalian reticuloendothelial system, stimulating the phagocytic activity of macrophages. When combined with antifungal drugs, it has provided satisfactory responses in the control of infections caused by pathogenic fungi.

In a refractory case of canine sporotrichosis caused by *Sporothrix brasiliensis*, the animal was only clinically cured of its lesion located in the nasal planum after four subcutaneous applications of (1-3)-β-glucan (0.5 mg/animal) every 7 days, in association with itraconazole (10 mg/kg) orally every 12 hours. Although few side effects have been reported with this therapy, granulomas may form in the areas applied, which subside in a few weeks without complications.

2.7.3. Thermotherapy

During pregnancy, the use of antifungal drugs is contraindicated in most cases, due to their potential embryotoxic and teratogenic effects. In these cases, patients can use daily thermotherapy, through the application of local heat by means of hot water bags at a temperature of around 40° to 43°C. The use of thermotherapy is recommended for small, localized lesions, especially in cutaneous and lymphocutaneous cases. In one feline, the disease was controlled by immersing the forelimb, containing a single lesion, in hot water at a temperature of 40°C, twice a day for 7 days.

Local heat helps in antifungal therapy, since *Sporothrix* spp. phagocytosed by defense cells showed a higher death rate when subjected to heat above 40°C compared to those phagocytosed and kept at 37°C. However, local thermotherapy is limited due to the fact that it depends on the location of the lesions, the correct time for its suspension and the difficulty in determining the appropriate temperature, as well as the animal's cooperation in the therapy.

CHAPTER 3

The Current Scenario of Sporotrichosis

Despite the therapeutic options that have been effectively adopted, recent studies have shown the existence of fungi from the *Sporothrix schenckii* complex that are resistant to the antifungal drugs used in clinical routine. The *Sporothrix brasiliensis* species seems to have a high genetic aptitude for generating new cells with different antifungal susceptibility profiles, and can generate clones capable of resisting the action of drugs.

Antifungal resistance has already been demonstrated in several *in vitro* studies and has alerted researchers and health professionals to the difficulty of controlling it. In recent clinical cases in dogs, cats and even humans, therapy with a single antifungal drug has failed to produce a satisfactory response, requiring an Increase in dose and even the combination of drugs with other agents in an attempt to control the disease. Although the molecular mechanisms involved in the process of antifungal resistance are little known, indiscriminate and negligent exposure to antifungals, as well as the interruption of treatment without medical/veterinary authorization, are one of the contributing factors to the emergence of antifungal-resistant strains *of Sporothrix* sp.

Faced with this current problem, we recognize the importance of correctly adopting therapeutic measures in human and animal patients in an attempt to control this disease. Furthermore, the need to research new active antifungal molecules is urgent, given the current situation.

CHAPTER 4

The Search for Therapeutic Alternatives

Faced with the problem of antifungal resistance, the search for promising molecules for the development of new antifungal drugs has been conducted scientifically through medicinal plants, which have biological properties of medical and veterinary interest. Around 80% of the world's population uses plants in different extractions and applications to meet their basic health needs. Many of these plants are studied and their active chemical compounds isolated for the preparation of medicines by the pharmaceutical industry.

These plants are recognized by the population by their popular names, which vary between geographic regions of the world, and there may even be the same name for different plants. To avoid misidentification, the genus and species of the plant must be known, which should be done in herbaria. Among the forms of medicinal use, different parts of the plants are used, such as roots, bark, leaves and/or combinations thereof, which are often prepared in the form of infusions, decoctions and macerations. Essential oils are also extracted and used as flavorings in the food industry, as well as pharmaceuticals, personal care products and perfumery.

In human and animal sporotrichosis, several studies have demonstrated the antifungal activity of different botanical species in different extraction preparations, with Lamiaceae, Combretaceae, Asteraceae and other botanical families being highlighted in this book.

4.1. Plants of the Lamiaceae Family

The Lamiaceae family is largely made up of aromatic herbs, shrubs and, occasionally, trees that generally have quadrangular branches. It comprises approximately 300 botanical genera and around 7500 plant species. Around the world, hundreds of species from this family are used as aromatic and medicinal plants, with basil, mint and sage being some of the herbs known by their popular names.

In general, plants of the Lamiaceae family are known for their extensive production of volatile compounds rich in biologically active substances of pharmaceutical interest, which constitute essential oils obtained from different parts of the plant, such as flowers, buds, seeds, leaves, branches, bark, wood, roots and even fruit.

Various biological properties are attributed to plants of the Lamiaceae family, which depend on the botanical species used. With regard to antimicrobial properties, various pathogens of medical and veterinary interest have been sensitive to different plants from this family *in in vitro* studies.

Plants of the genera *Ocimum* spp. (popularly known as alfavaca, basil) and the species *Origanum vulgare* (oregano) and *O. majorana* (marjoram), *Rosmarinus officinalis* (rosemary) and *Salvia lavanduloides* (sage) have been one of the outstanding plants *in the* Lamiaceae family with proven *in vitro* activity against fungi of the *Sporothrix schenckii* complex.

4.1.1. *Ocimum* spp.

Ocimum spp. are popularly known as alfavaca, alfavaca-cravo, manjericâo, and other synonyms, due to their botanical similarities. Widely distributed in tropical and warm climate regions, plants of the genus *Ocimum* spp. are often used for therapeutic purposes, as antitussives and in respiratory disorders, as well as against headaches, kidney and gastrointestinal disorders, including those caused by bacteria.

Antifungal activity has been demonstrated in ethanolic extracts of *O. gratissum* leaves from Nigeria against *Malassezia furfur* and dermatophytes. In *O. sanctum* leaves from India, aqueous and alcoholic extracts and different fractions, such as hexane, benzene, chloroform and ethyl acetate, were active against *E. floccosum, M. gypseum, M. nanum, T. mentagrophytes* and *T. rubrum*.

Although studies on fungi from the *Sporothrix schenckii* complex are scarce, the essential oils of *O. basilicum* (Figure 6), *O. canum* (synonym *of O. americanum*), *O. gratissimum* and *O. sanctum* from India have inhibited the growth of *S. schenckii* using the agar-diffusion technique, where inhibition of fungal growth was observed in a halo between 8 and 14 mm in diameter. However, the ethanolic extract of *Ocimum micranthum* leaves showed no activity against *S. schenckii* when tested at the maximum concentration of 0.2 mg/mL for both dimorphic phases of the fungal agent.

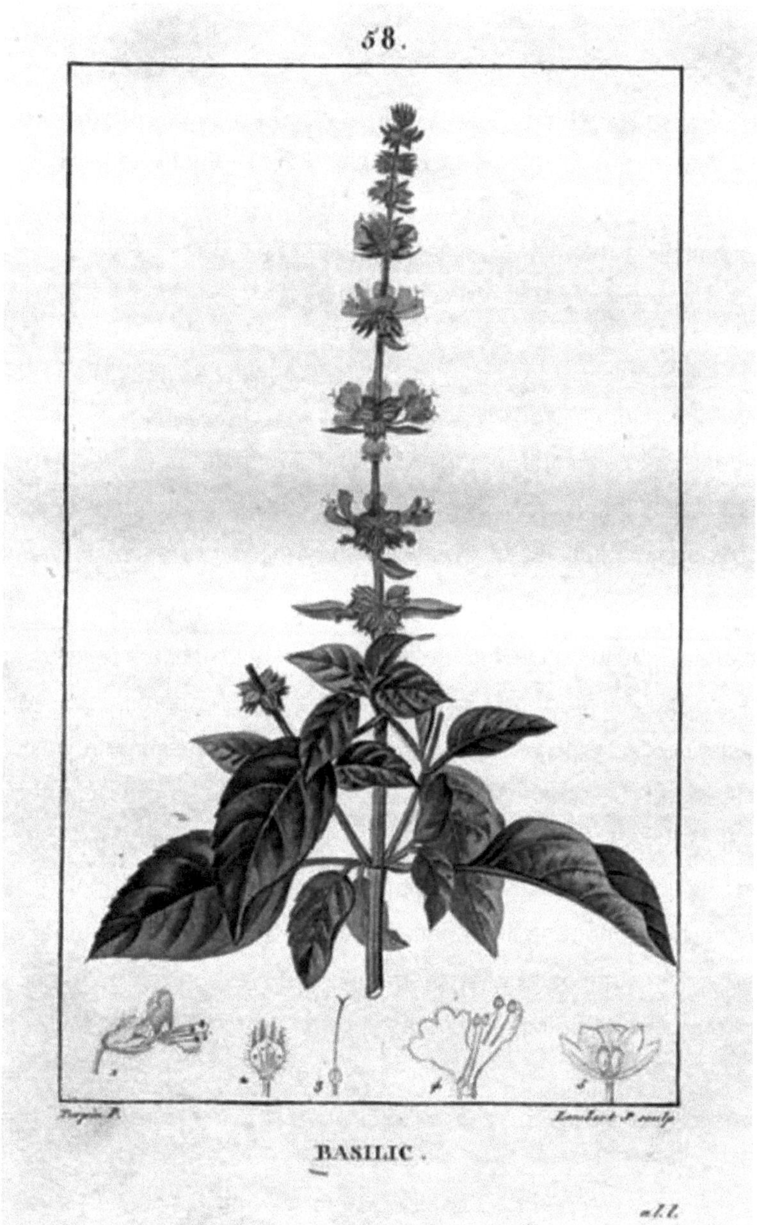

Figure 6 - Anatomical illustration of *Ocimum basilicum,* from the Lamiaceae/Labiateae family (CHAUMETON, 1833), which had *in vitro* activity against *S. schenckii.*

4.1.2. *Origanum* spp.

In *Origanum* spp., two botanical species have stood out as promising candidates for the development of possible drugs against *Sporothrix* spp., these being *O. vulgare* and *O. majorana*. Both plants are aromatic herbs widely used in cooking and have potential therapeutic applications, especially as they produce essential oils with antimicrobial properties.

4.1.2.1. *Origanum vulgare*

Popularly used for its antispasmodic, carminative and antiseptic properties, the botanical species *Origanum vulgare* is known as oregano (Figure 7) and is used as a sudorifera to stimulate perspiration and sweating, as well as for its tonic properties. Its antifungal properties have been demonstrated mainly with its essential oils against species of *Candida* spp., *Malassezia pachydermatis* and *S. schenckii* and *S. brasiliensis.*

At concentrations of 250 to 500 µL/mL, the essential oil of *O. vulgare* from Chile inhibited *S. schenckii* isolated from cats and humans with sporotrichosis. In studies with standard strains and clinical isolates of human sporotrichosis, oregano oil inhibited *S. schenckii* (MIC of 216.8 to 1735 µg/mL) and *S.* brasiliensis (MIC of 1735 µg/mL). *brasiliensis* (MIC from 433.7 to 867.5 µg/mL), this variation in antifungal activity being attributed to the morphological changes they cause in the fungal hyphae and the reduction in the number of adhered conidia. The compound γ-terpinene has been recognized as a major component of oregano essential oil and has shown *in vitro* efficacy at MICs of between 62.5 and 500 µg/mL for *S. schenckii* and between 125 and 250 µg/mL for *S. brasiliensis*.

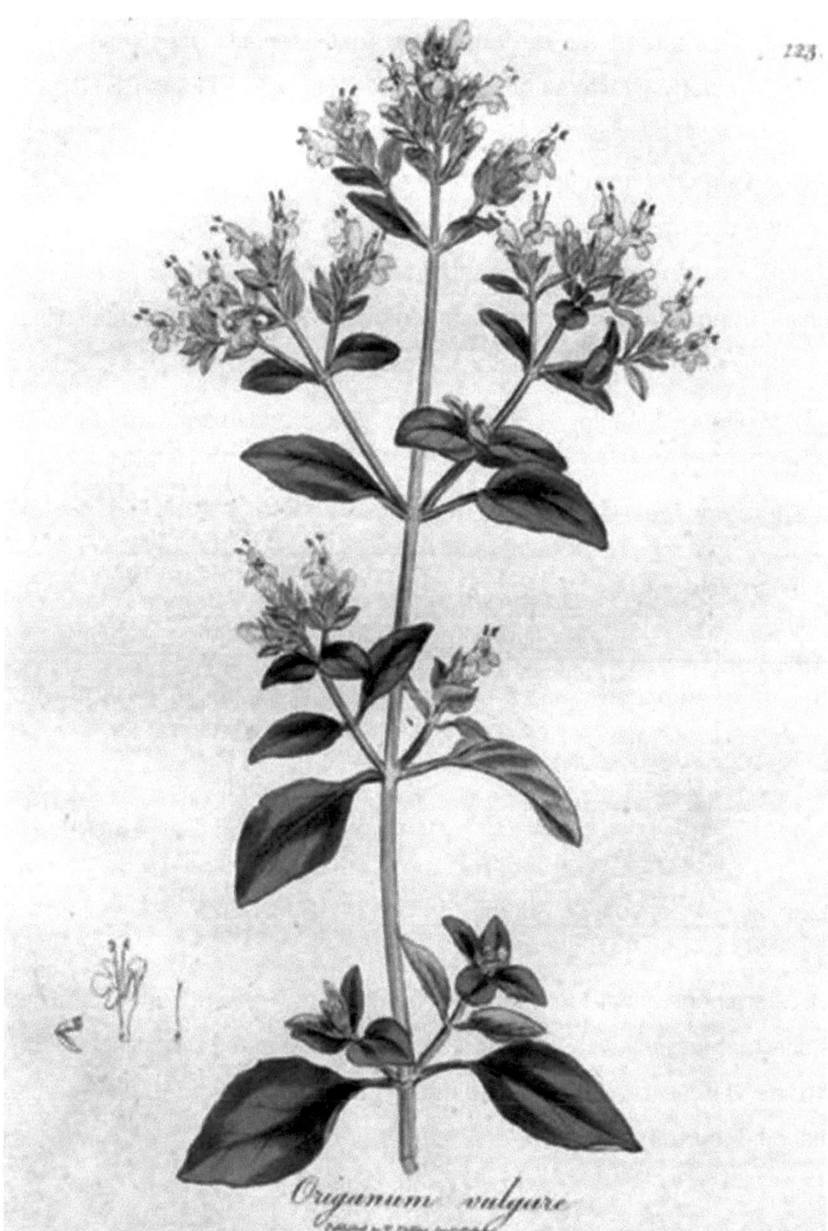

Figura 7. Anatomical illustration of *Origanum vulgare* Linn., from the Lamiaceae family (WOODVILLE, 1832), with potential activity against *Sporothrix schenckii* and *Sporothrix brasiliensis*.

In recent studies carried out by the Center for Diagnosis and Research in Veterinary Mycology (Universidade Federal de Pelotas, Pelotas/RS, Brazil), the yeast phase of *S. brasiliensis* isolated from dogs and cats was sensitive to essential oil extracted from aerial parts of *O. vulgare aerial parts* collected in Chile and the commercial oil from Moldavia at MICs of ≤2.25 to 9 mg/mL and ≤2.25 to 36 mg/mL, respectively, including against itraconazole-resistant *S. brasiliensis*. Fungicidal activity was also demonstrated by both essential oils at concentrations similar to the fungistatic ones (Table 1).

Table 1. Minimum inhibitory concentration (MIC) and minimum fungicidal concentration (MFC) of extracted and commercial essential oils of *O. vulgare* against *Sporothrix brasiliensis* and *S. schenckii*.

Fungal origin (No. of samples)		***Origanum vulg* Extract**		*rare* **(oregano)* Commercial**	
		CIM	**CFM**	**CIM**	**CFM**
S. brasiliensis					
Cats (8)	Variation	≤2,25 - 9	≤2,25 - 9	≤2,25 - 18	≤2,25 - 36
	50%	≤2,25	≤2,25	9	9
	90%	4,5	4,5	18	18
Dogs (6)	Variation	≤2,25	≤2,25 - 4,5	≤2,25 - 36	≤2,25 - 36
	50%	≤2,25	≤2,25	≤2,25	4,5
	90%	≤2,25	≤2,25	9	18
S. schenckii					
IOC 1226 (1)	Variation	≤2,25	≤2,25	≤2,25	≤2,25

*Results expressed in mg/mL.

Thymol, α-terpinene and 4-terpineol have been the major compounds identified by gas chromatography with flame ionization detector in the oil extracted from oregano, as well as carvacrol, γ-terpinene and *p-cymene* in the commercial essential oil (Figure 8).

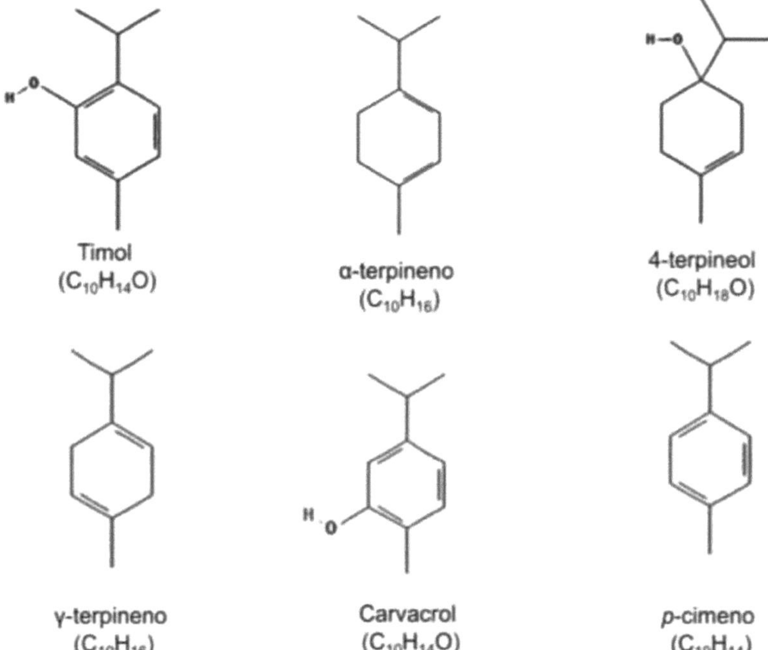

Figura 8. Chemical structural representation of the major compounds of *Origanum vulgare* found in the extracted (Chile) - thymol, α-terpinene and 4- terpineol - and commercial (Moldavia) essential oils - carvacrol, γ-terpinene and *p-cymene* - and their respective molecular formulas.

These chemical compounds have aromatic rings in their structural composition, which the polar group contained in these rings allows hydrogen bonding to the active sites of target microbial enzymes, allowing increased permeability of the fungal cytoplasmic membrane and consequent destruction of its physical structure, which is reflected in the antifungal activity of these compounds.

In addition, the leakage of cytoplasmic contents caused by these chemical compounds promotes the depletion of ergosterol, which is the steroid component essential for the proper functioning of the fungal cell membrane.

The difference observed in the chromatographic chemical composition would explain why the extracted essential oil has shown better *anti-Sporothrix* spp.

activity *in vitro* compared to the commercial essential oil of *O. vulgare*, and would be due to various factors related to the plant, such as place and time of cultivation, type of climate and soil, botanical genetics, harvesting method, among others.

4.1.2.2. *Origanum majorana*

Origanum majorana is used in folk medicine for its sedative, antitussive, antispasmodic and diuretic properties, as well as for its use against colic, dizziness, migraines and headaches. Infusions of *O. majorana* are also used to relieve signs of asthma and for their sudorific and menstrual flow (emmenagogue) and lactation (lactogogue) stimulating activities in women. Several fungal pathogens have shown sensitivity to *O. majorana* essential oil, such as *Malassezia pachydermatis* and the dermatophytes *E. floccosum, M. canis, M. gypseum, T. mentagrophytes, T. rubrum* and *T. tonsurans.*

Candida albicans has been sensitive to methanolic extracts of *O. majorana,* as have the anemophilic fungi *Fusarium solani, Aspergillus niger, A. parasiticus, Rhizopus oryzae, R. oryzae-sativae* and *Alternaria brassicicola*. These fungi are important in human health because they are airborne contaminants and promote opportunistic infections in the respiratory system of patients with weakened immunity or who are highly disposed to the propagules of these fungal microorganisms, which manifest allergic signs such as asthma and rhinitis.

In fungi of the *Sporothrix schenckii* complex, studies with *O. majorana* are scarce. Recently, *O. majorana* (Figure 9) has been shown to be promising for the development of antifungal drugs. The essential oil extracted from the aerial parts of the plant grown in Egypt has been shown to have fungistatic and fungicidal activities at MICs of ≤2.25 to 9 mg/mL and CFMs of ≤2.25 to 18 mg/mL (Table 2).

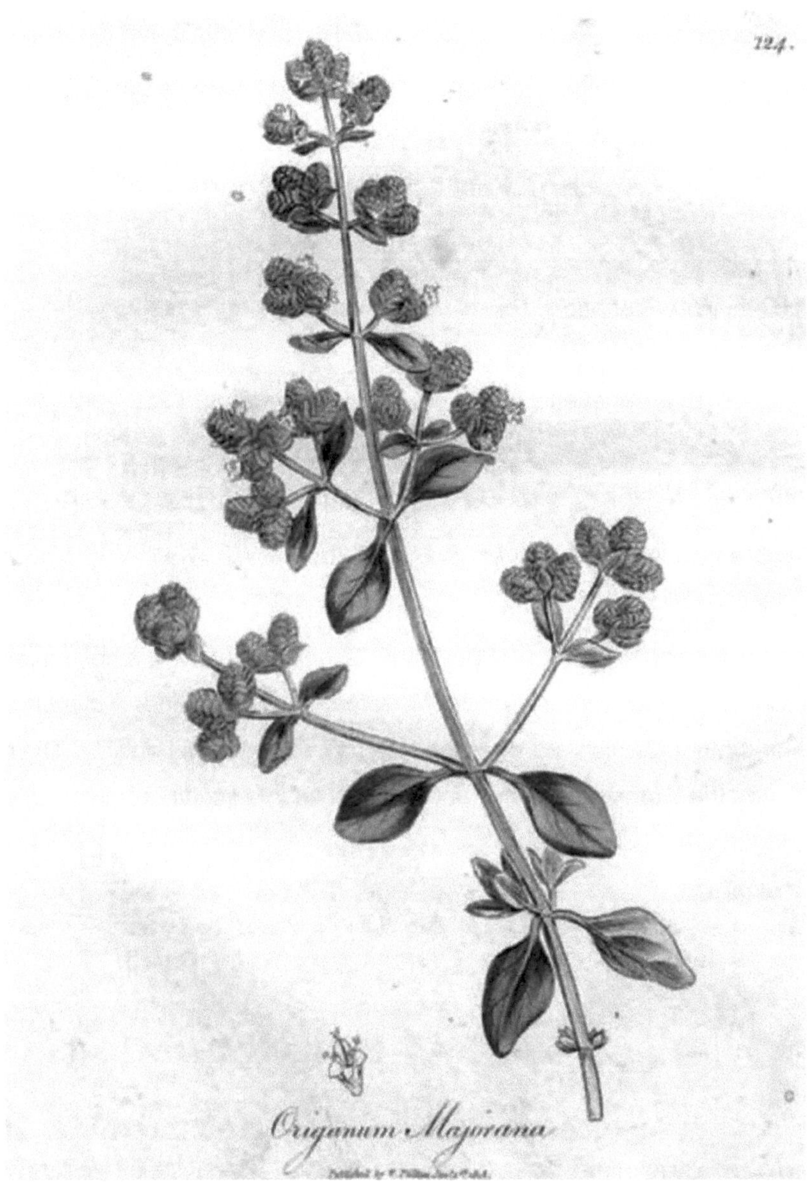

Figura 9. Anatomical illustration of *Origanum majorana* Linn., from the Lamiaceae family (WOODVILLE et al., 1832), which was active against *Sporothrix brasiliensis* and *Sporothrix schenckii*.

Table 2. Minimum inhibitory concentration (MIC) and minimum fungicidal concentration (MFC) of the commercial essential oil of *O. majorana* against *Sporothrix brasiliensis* and *S. schenckii*.

Fungal origin (No. of samples)		***Origanum majora* Coi oil**	***na* (marjoram)* nercial**
		CIM	**CFM**
S. brasiliensis			
Cats (8)	Variation	≤2,25 - 9	≤2,25 - 9
	50%	≤2,25	4,5
	90%	4,5	9
Dogs (6)	Variation	≤2,25 - 4,5	≤2,25 - 19
	50%	≤2,25	4,5
	90%	≤2,25	9
S. schenckii			
IOC 1226 (1)	Variation	≤2,25	≤2,25

*Results expressed in mg/mL.

Of the 22 chemical compounds identified in marjoram essential oil with anti-Sporothrix *brasiliensis* and anti-Sporothrix *schenckii* activity, the major substances recognized were 1,8-cineol, 4- terpineol, γ-terpinene, *p-cymene*, sabinene and others, which are described as having antifungal activity. Their chemical structural representations and respective molecular formulas are shown in Figure 10.

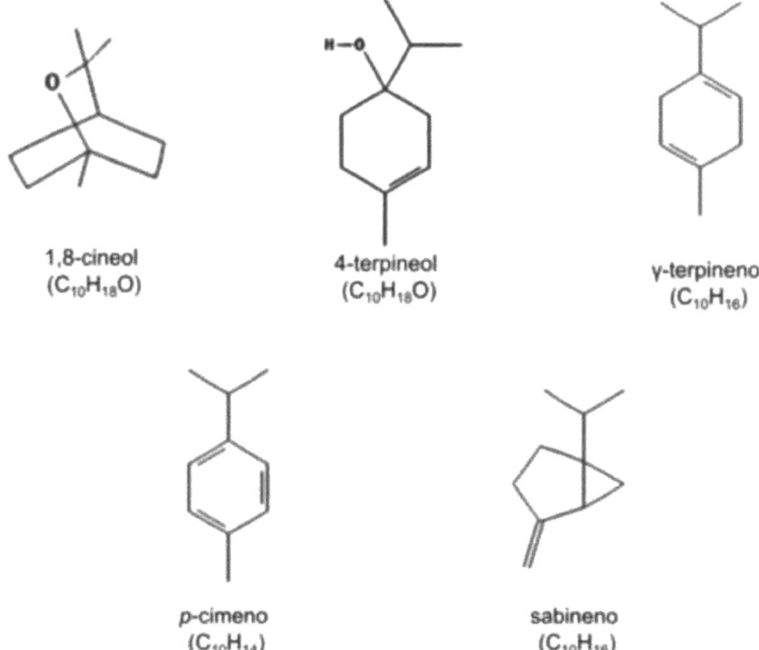

Figura 10. Chemical structural representation of the major compounds found in the commercial essential oil of *Origanum majorana* (Egypt) - 1,8-cineol, 4-terpineol, γ-terpinene, *p-cymene* and sabinene.

4.1.3. *Rosmarinus officinalis*

An aromatic herb often used in cooking and popularly known as rosemary, the species *Rosmarinus officinalis* (Figure 11) is used in traditional medicine for its respiratory, carminative, digestive and diuretic properties, as well as for rheumatic ailments and headaches.

The antifungal activity of *R. officinalis* has been attributed to its essential oil, since various pathogenic fungi have shown sensitivity *in vitro*, such as *Candida albicans*, *Cryptococcus neoformans*, *Epydermophyton floccosum*, *Trichophyton mentagrophytes*, *T. rubrum*, *Microsporum canis* and *M. gypseum*.

On *S. schenckii*, the minimum inhibitory concentration of the essential oil extracted from the aerial parts of *R. officinalis* collected in India was 11 mg/mL, and no fungicidal activity was observed at this maximum concentration tested by researchers in India.

Essential oils from different sources have been active *in vitro* against *S. brasiliensis* isolated from dogs and cats. In the essential oil extracted from aerial parts collected in Chile, *S. brasiliensis* was inhibited at MICs of ≤2.25 to 18 mg/mL, while fungicidal activity was conferred at CFMs of ≤2.25 to 72 mg/mL. In the essential oil obtained commercially and originating in Tunisia, activity was observed at MICs of ≤2.25 to 18 mg/mL and CFMs of ≤2.25 to >72 mg/mL. In the study, *S. schenckii* was more sensitive to the extracted essential oil (Table 3).

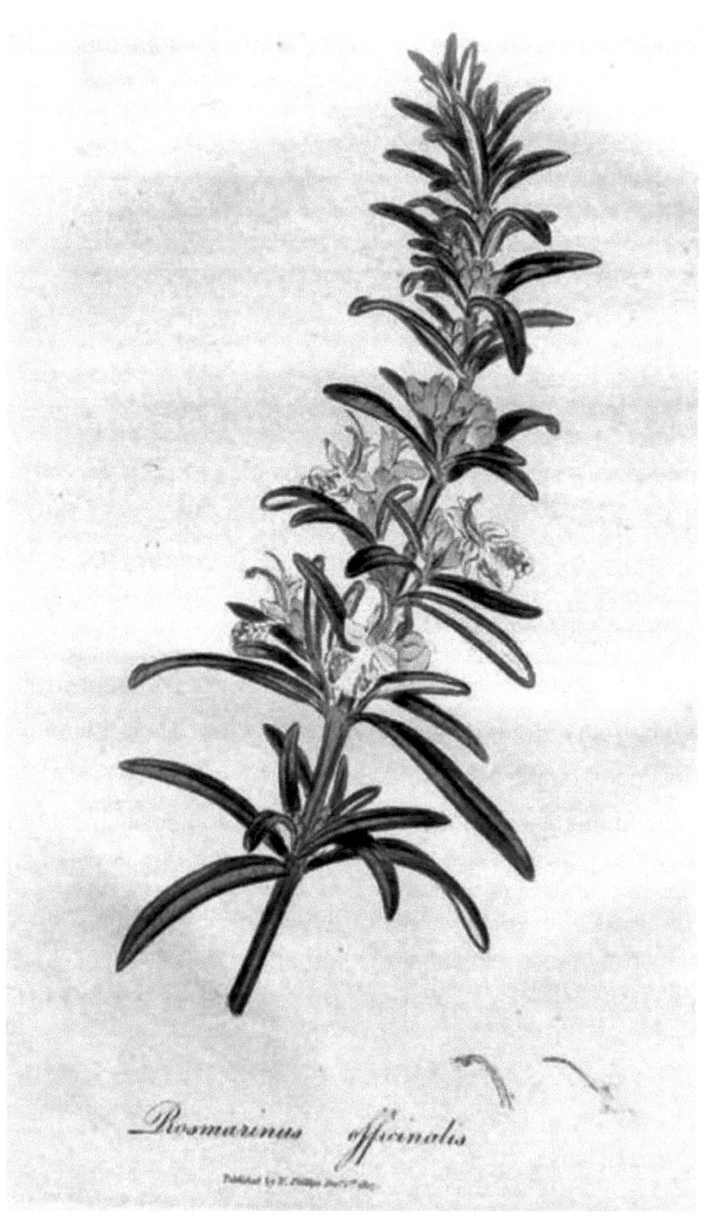

Figura 11. Anatomical illustration of *Rosmarinus officinalis* Linn., from the Lamiaceae family (WOODVILLE et al., 1832), which was active against *Sporothrix schenckii* and *Sporothrix brasiliensis*.

Table 3. Minimum inhibitory concentration (MIC) and minimum fungicidal concentration (MFC) of extracted and commercial essential oils of *R. officinalis* against *Sporothrix brasiliensis* and *S. schenckii*.

Fungal origin (No. of samples)	-	***Rosmarinus officialis* (rosemary)** Extracted		Commercial	
		CIM	**CFM**	**CIM**	**CFM**
S. brasiliensis					
Cats (8)	Variation	≤2,25 - 18	≤2,25 - 72	≤2,25 - 9	≤2,25 - 9
	50%	≤2,25	≤2,25	≤2,25	4,5
	90%	18	36	4,5	4,5
Dogs (6)	Variation	≤2,25	≤2,25 - 4,5	≤2,25 - 18	4,5 - >72
	50%	≤2,25	≤2,25	4,5	9
	90%	≤2,25	4,5	18	36
S. schenckii					
IOC1226 (1)	Variation	≤2,25	≤2,25	18	36

*Results expressed in mg/mL.

Both essential oils of *R. officinalis* were analyzed by gas chromatography with flame ionization detector and showed similar chemical composition. Although a total of 12 chemical compounds were detected in the extracted essential oil and at least 19 in the commercial essential oil, the majority composition of both products showed the presence of 1,8-cineole and α-pinene for both, followed by camphene for the oil extracted in Chile and camphor for the commercial oil from Tunisia, as shown by the chemical structures and respective molecular formulas (Figure 12).

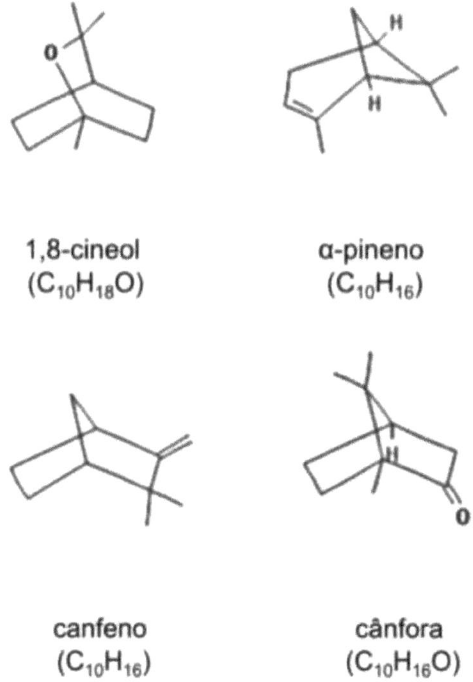

Figura 12. Chemical structural representation of the major compounds of *Rosmarinus officinalis* found in the extracted essential oil (Chile) - 1,8-cineol, α-pinene and camphene - and commercial essential oil (Tunisia) - 1,8-cineol, camphor and α-pinene - and their respective molecular formulas.

The compounds 1,8-cineole and α-pinene have antibacterial and antifungal activity against various pathogens of medical and veterinary interest. As they are major components of both oils, the presence of these compounds seems to be important in conferring their antifungal activity, since the inhibition of growth and death of *S. brasiliensis* and *S. schenckii* was observed in a similar way for both secondary metabolites of these plants.

4.1.4. *Salvia lavanduloides*

The genus *Salvia* spp. comprises around 900 species, which are mainly found in the Mediterranean, southeast Africa and Central and South America and are widely cultivated for medicinal, culinary and ornamental use. *Salvia lavanduloides* is an aromatic plant widely distributed in Central America and southern Mexico and is used in folk medicine for its antiseptic, healing, anti-inflammatory and antirheumatic properties.

The antimicrobial activity of *Salvia* spp. has been reported and attributed to the major compounds in its essential oils, such as 1,8-cineole, camphor, borneol, *p-cymene*, α-thujone, among others.

Few studies have been carried out on the genus *Salvia* spp. against pathogenic fungi that cause sporotrichosis. Clinical isolates of *S. schenckii* from humans were tested against the ethanolic extract of *S. lavanduloides* leaves and flowers collected in Guatemala at a MIC of 0.5 mg/mL for the yeast phase, while the mycelial phase showed no sensitivity *in vitro*. However, when tested at the maximum concentration of 100 μg/mL, the same type of extract showed no efficacy against *S. schenckii.*

4.2. Plants of the Combretaceae Family

The Combretaceae family comprises about 18 botanical genera, with *Combretum* spp. representing at least 370 species and *Terminalia* spp. with about 200 species, which are plants widely distributed in West and South Africa. In different regions of the African continent, several species of plants from the Combretaceae family are used by traditional peoples for medicinal purposes, such as the treatment of gastrointestinal disorders such as diarrhea and dysentery, urinary disorders, cardiac disorders and respiratory disorders such as coughs, colds and pneumonia. It has also been used for sore throats, back pain, ear and throat pain, fever and general weakness, among other ailments.

The antimicrobial activities of Combretaceae plants have been investigated and proven, especially in relation to the antibacterial activity of *Terminalia* sp. species. In pathogenic fungi, the antifungal activity of different *Terminalia* spp. species against *Candida albicans, Cryptococcus neoformans, Aspergillus fumigatus, Microsporum canis* and also against *Sporothrix schenckii* has been observed.

Isolates of *S. schenckii* have been sensitive to acetonic, hexanic, dichloromethanic and methanolic extracts prepared from the fresh leaves of the trees *Terminalia prunioides, T. brachystemma, T. sericea, T. gazensis, T. mollis* and *T. sambesiaca* native to South Africa at MICs ranging from 0.02 to 0.64 mg/mL (Table 4).

Table 4 Botanical species of the Combretaceae family and their active extracts with *in vitro* inhibitory activity against *Sporothrix schenckii.*

Botanical species	Extract t	Minimum inhibitory concentration (mg/mL)
Combretum* spp.		
C. acutifolium	Ac, He, Di, Me	0,04 a 0,32
C. albopunctactum	Ac, He, Di, Me	0,08 a 0,32
C. apiculatum spp. *apiculatum*	Ac, He, Di, Me	0,02 a 0,04
C. bracteosum	Ac, He, Di, Me	0,08 a 0,16
C. caffrum	Ac, He, Di, Me	0,32 a 0,64
C. celastroides spp. *celastroids*	Ac, He, Di, Me	0,16 a 0,32
C. celastroides spp. *oriental*	Ac, He, Di, Me	0,08 a 0,16
C. collinum spp. *suluense*	Ac, He, Di, Me	0,16 a 2,5
C. collinum spp. *taborense*	Ac, He, Di, Me	0,32 a 0,64
C. edwardsii	Ac, He, Di, Me	0,04 a 0,08
C. erythrophyllum	He, Di, Me	0,32 a 1,25
C. hereroense	Ac, He, Di, Me	0,16 a 0,32
C. imberbe	Di	0,32
C. kraussii	Ac, He, Di, Me	0,32 a 0,64
C. microphyllum	Ac, He, Di, Me	0,32 a 0,64
C. moggii	Ac, He, Di, Me	0,02 a 0,16
C. molle	Ac, He, Di, Me	0,08 a 0,32
C. mossambicense	Ac, He, Di, Me	0,16 a 0,64
C. nelsonii	Ac, He, Di, Me	0,08 a 0,32
C. padoides	Ac, Me	0,32 a 0,64
C. paniculatum	Ac, He, Di, Me	0,04 a 0,32
C. petrophilum	Ac, He, Di, Me	0,04 a 0,32
C. woodii	Ac, He, Di, Me	0,32 a 1,25
C. zeyheri	Ac, He, Di, Me	0,02 a 0,08
*C. vendae***	He	0,13
Terminalia* spp.**		

T. brachystemma	Ac, He, Di, Me	0,32 a 0,64
T. gazensis	Ac, He, Di, Me	0,08 a 0,16
T. mollis	Ac, He, Di, Me	0,02 a 0,16
T. prunioides	Ac, He, Di, Me	0,32 a 0,64
T. sambesiaca	Ac, He, Di, Me	0,02 a 0,16
T. sericeae	Ac, He, Di, Me	0,32 a 0,64

* Masoko et al. (2007); ** Suleiman et al. (2009); *** Masoko et al.(2005);

t Ac - acetone; He - hexane; Di - dichloromethane; Me - methanol;

In *Combretum* spp., 24 plant species from this genus were tested against *S. schenckii* isolated from a horse with cutaneous lymphangitis using the broth microdilution technique. The results showed that all the plant extracts had inhibitory activity at concentrations of 0.02 to 0.32 mg/mL, with *C. zeyheri* standing out (Figure 13), which inhibited at MICs of 0.02 to 0.08 mg/mL. *Combretum vendae* also inhibited *S. schenckii* at an MIC of 0.13 mg/mL.

In studies with animals experimentally infected with different fungal pathogens, including *S. schenckii*, the acetone extracts prepared from the leaves of *Combretum imberbe, C. nelsonii*, *C. albopunctatum* and *Terminalia sericea* proved to be effective in the healing process of wounds when prepared at 20% (2g of extract/10g of cream) and administered topically three times a week to Wistar rats. The wounds were clinically reversed in at least 15 days of treatment, with no apparent adverse effects, indicating the promising use of the extract in antifungal treatment.

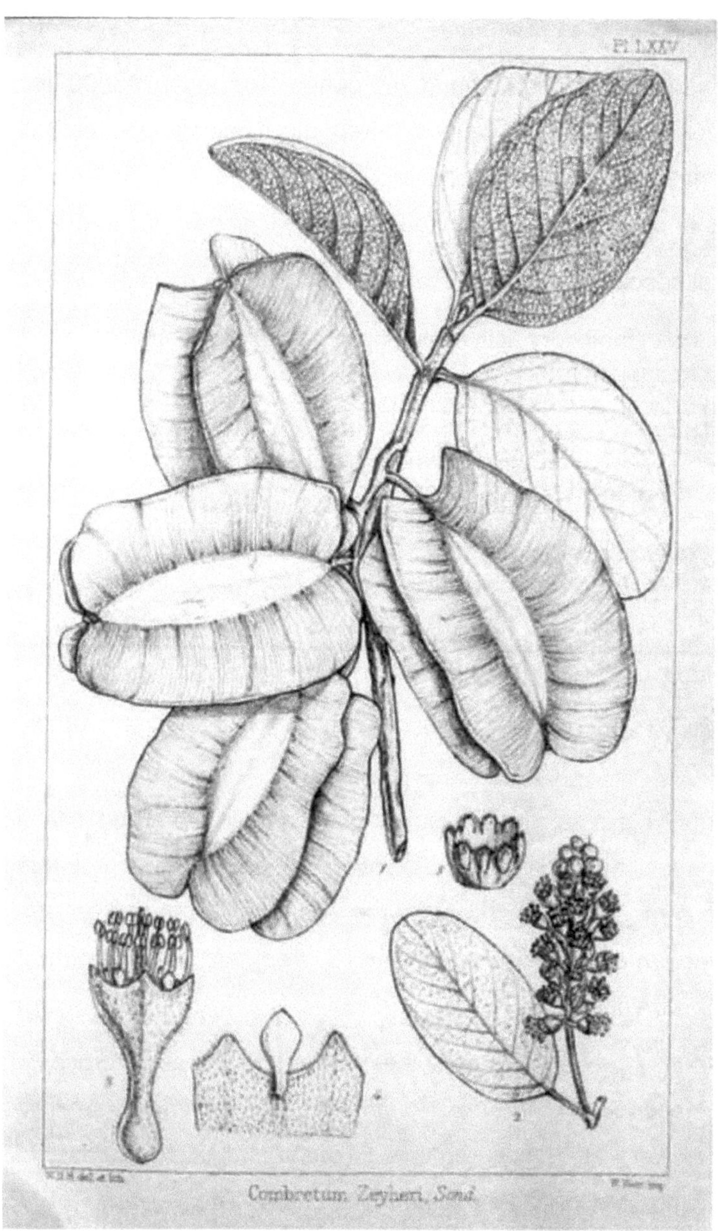

Figure 13. Anatomical illustration of *Combretum zeyheri* Sonder., from the Combretaceae family (HARVEY, 1859), one of the South African botanical species with potential activity against *S. schenckii*.

4.3. Plants of the Asteraceae Family

The Asteraceae family comprises around 380 genera with at least 3000 plant species, which are known for their various therapeutic, cosmetic and aromatic properties. Information on the *in vitro* antifungal susceptibility of *S. schenckii* to different extracts of plants from the Asteraceae family is shown in Table 5.

Table 5 Botanical species of the Asteraceae family and their extracts active ingredients with inhibitory activity against *Sporothrix schenckii.*

Botanical species	Anatomical part	Extract*	Reference
Artemisia ludoviciana	Leaves, Flowers, Roots	EA, MC	a
Heliopsis longipes	Leaves, Flowers, Roots	Aq, EA, MC	a
Ophryosporus peruvianus	Leaves, Stems	E	b
Pterocaulon balansae	Aerial parts	Me	c
Pterocaulon cordobense	Aerial parts	Me	c
Pterocaulon lanatum	Aerial parts	Me	c
Pterocaulon lorentzii	Aerial parts	Me	c
Pterocaulon polystachyum	Aerial parts	Me	c
Senecio culcitioides	Aerial parts	E	b
Tagetes lucida	Leaves, Flowers, Roots	Aq, EA, MC	a

*Aq - aqueous; EA - ethyl acetate; MC - methanol-chloroform; E - ethanol; Me - methanol. [a] Damiân-Badillo *et al.*, 2008; b Rojas *et al.*, 2003; c Stopiglia *et al.*, 2011

Among the plants in this family that stand out for their promising use as antifungals, the species of the genus *Pterocaulon* spp. showed properties against *Microsporum gypseum, Trichophyton rubrum, T. mentagrophytes, Cryptococcus neoformans, Candida albicans, C. tropicalis, Saccharomyces cerevisiae* and *S. schenckii.*

Methanolic extracts prepared from the aerial parts of *Pterocaulon polystachyum*, *P. balansae, P. lorentzii, P. lanatum* and *P. cordobense* native to southern Brazil were also active against 24 human clinical isolates of *S. schenckii*, including itraconazole-resistant isolates. The extract of *P. polystachyum* (Figure 14) was shown to have high antifungal activity, since it presented the best MIC values between 156 and 312 µg/mL. The other species of *Pterocaulon* spp. tested were active with MICs between 156 and 1250 µg/mL.

In *Peruvian* folk medicine, *Ophryosporus peruvianus* is a plant commonly used as an antiseptic and to treat skin wounds. *Senecio culcitioides* is often used to treat coughs, asthma and respiratory problems. Both plants were studied by researchers in Peru, who observed the inhibitory activity of ethanolic extracts of the leaves and stems of *Ophryosporus peruvianus* and aerial parts of *Senecio culcitioides* against *S. schenckii*, inhibited by 13 mm and 15 mm respectively. These studies showed the sensitivity of other pathogenic fungi of veterinary medical importance, such as *Candida albicans* and *Trichophyton mentagrophytes*, although the dermatophyte *Microsporum gypseum* was not sensitive.

In plants native to Mexico, the extracts of different anatomical parts of *Artemisia ludoviciana, Heliopsis longipes* and *Tagetes lucida* (Figure 15) were active against *S. schenckii*. These plants are commonly used in folk medicine in different countries for their biological properties, including antimicrobial properties. For these plants, the preparation of the extract using ethyl acetate or methanol-chloroform showed better activity against *S. schenckii* than the preparation of the aqueous extract, demonstrating that the type of solvent can influence the antifungal activity of the same plant.

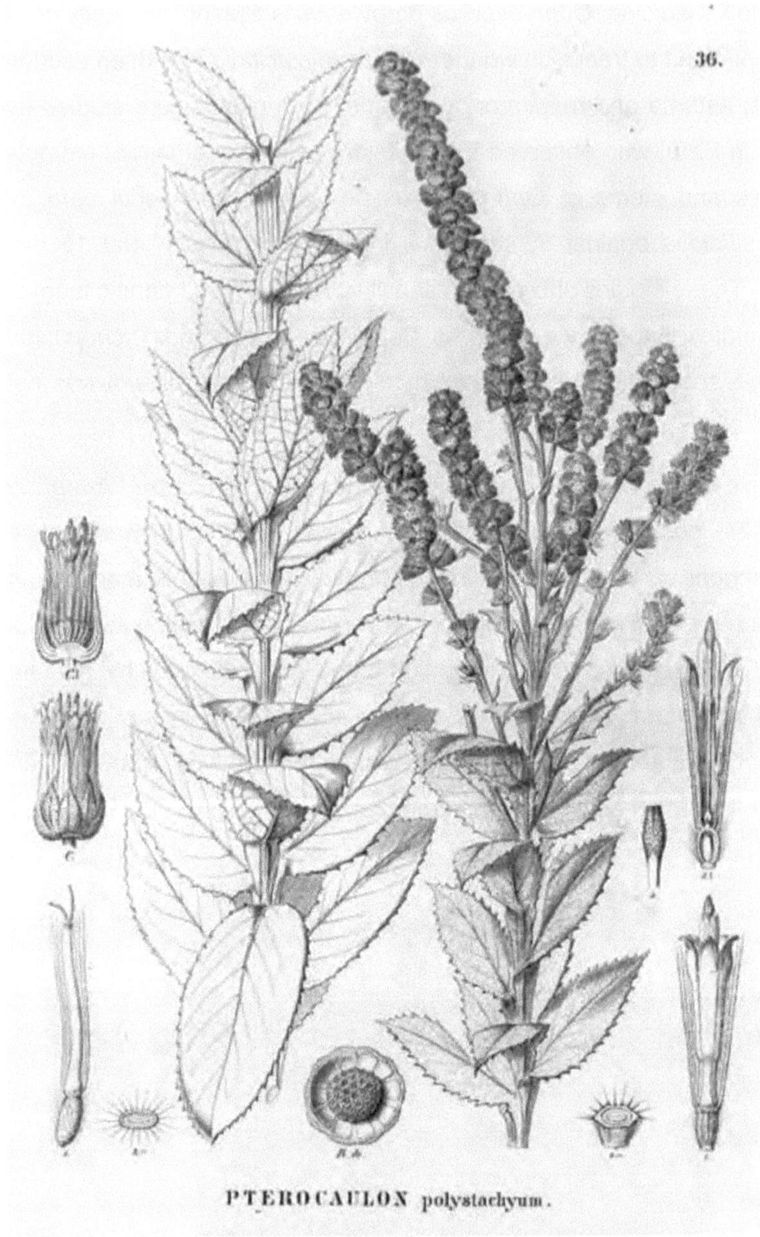

Figura 14. Anatomical illustration of *Pterocaulon polystachyum,* from the Asteraceae family (MARTIUS et al., 1882), with anti-Sporothrix *schenckii* potential.

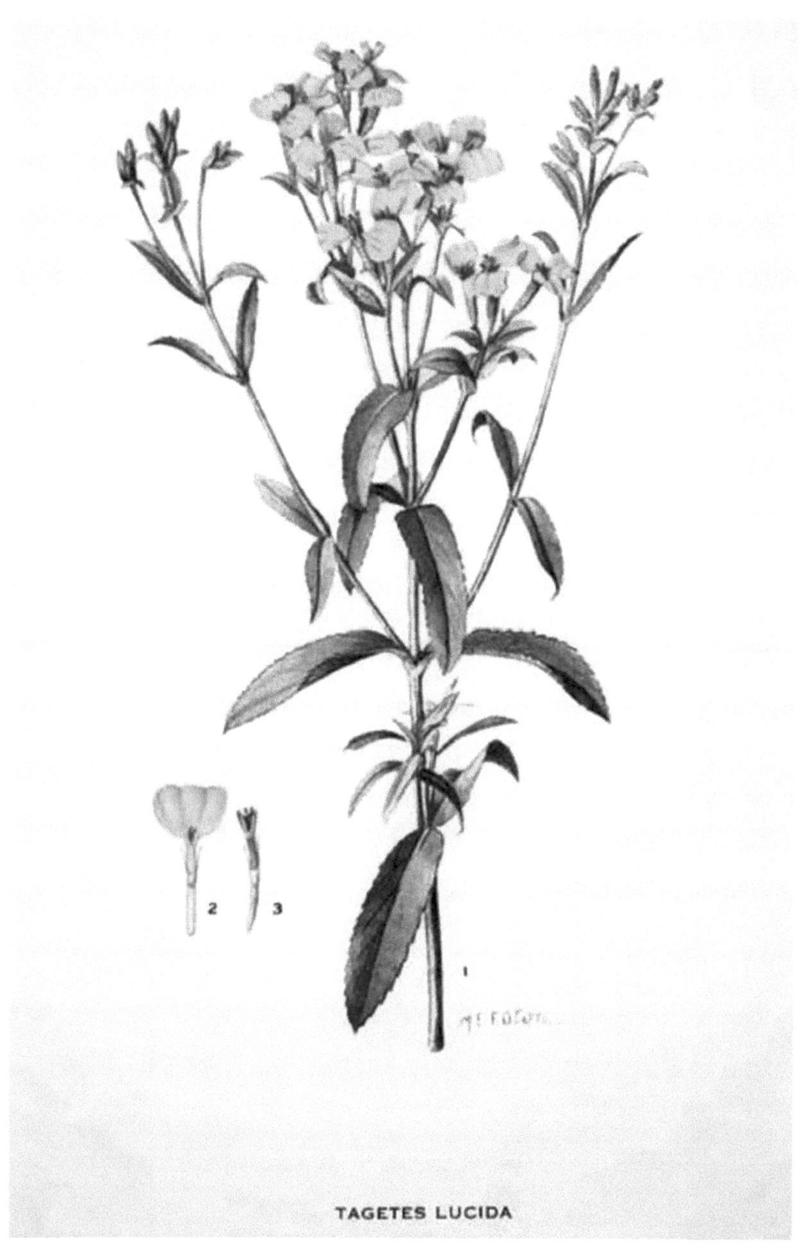

Figura 15. Anatomical illustration of *Tagetes lucida* Cav., from the Asteraceae family (EATON, 1931), which showed activity against *S. schenckii*.

4.4. Plants of the Myrtaceae Family

The plants of the Myrtaceae family have around 3,000 species belonging to around 150 botanical genera, and are widely distributed in regions of the world with a warm, tropical climate. Due to their fragrance and flavoring potential, many of these species are used to produce essential oils, which have been shown to have various biological properties, including antifungal properties.

In the *Eucalyptus* spp. genus, the inhibitory activity on the growth of *S. schenckii* was observed in the 12 mm zone for the acetone extract of the leaves of the *E. Camaldulensis* trees (Figure 16), which originated in Mexico, as well as the essential oil of the leaves of the *E. Citriodora* tree from India, which inhibited up to the 27 mm zone.

In fruit trees of the *Psidium* spp. genus, the methanolic extracts of the leaves of *Psidium guajava* (Figure 17), popularly known as guava, caused a 16 mm zone of inhibition against *S. sChenCkii*. The ethanolic extracts of the leaves of *P. aCutangulum*, collected in Peru and popularly known in Brazil as araçandiba or araçâ-pera, inhibited *S. schenckii* by 22 mm. Another plant from the Myrtaceae family with antifungal potential was *Syzygium aromaticum*, known as clove, in which *S. schenckii* was inhibited in 43 mm of zone by the hexanic extract of the buds of the flowers of this tree.

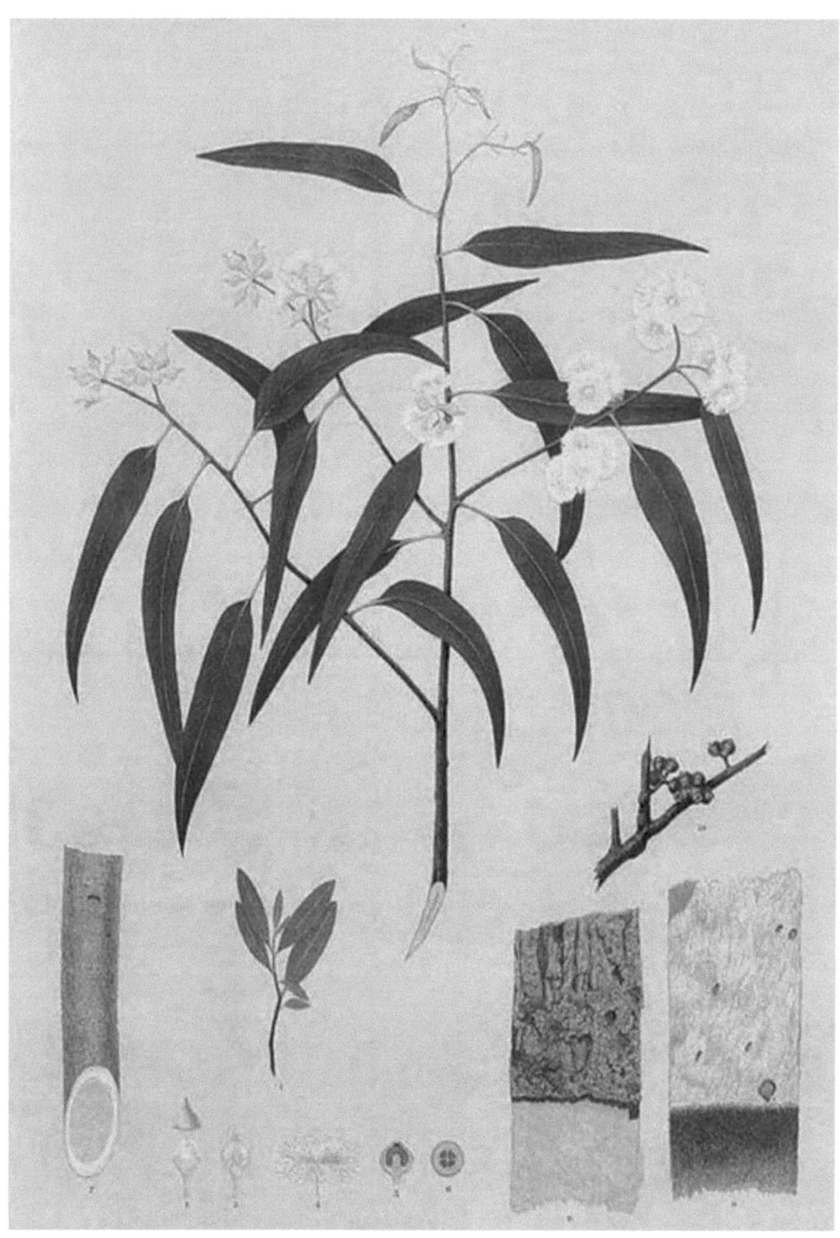

Figura 16. Anatomical illustration of *Eucalyptus Camaldulensis,* from the Myrtaceae family (BROWN, 1833), which showed activity against *S. schenckii.*

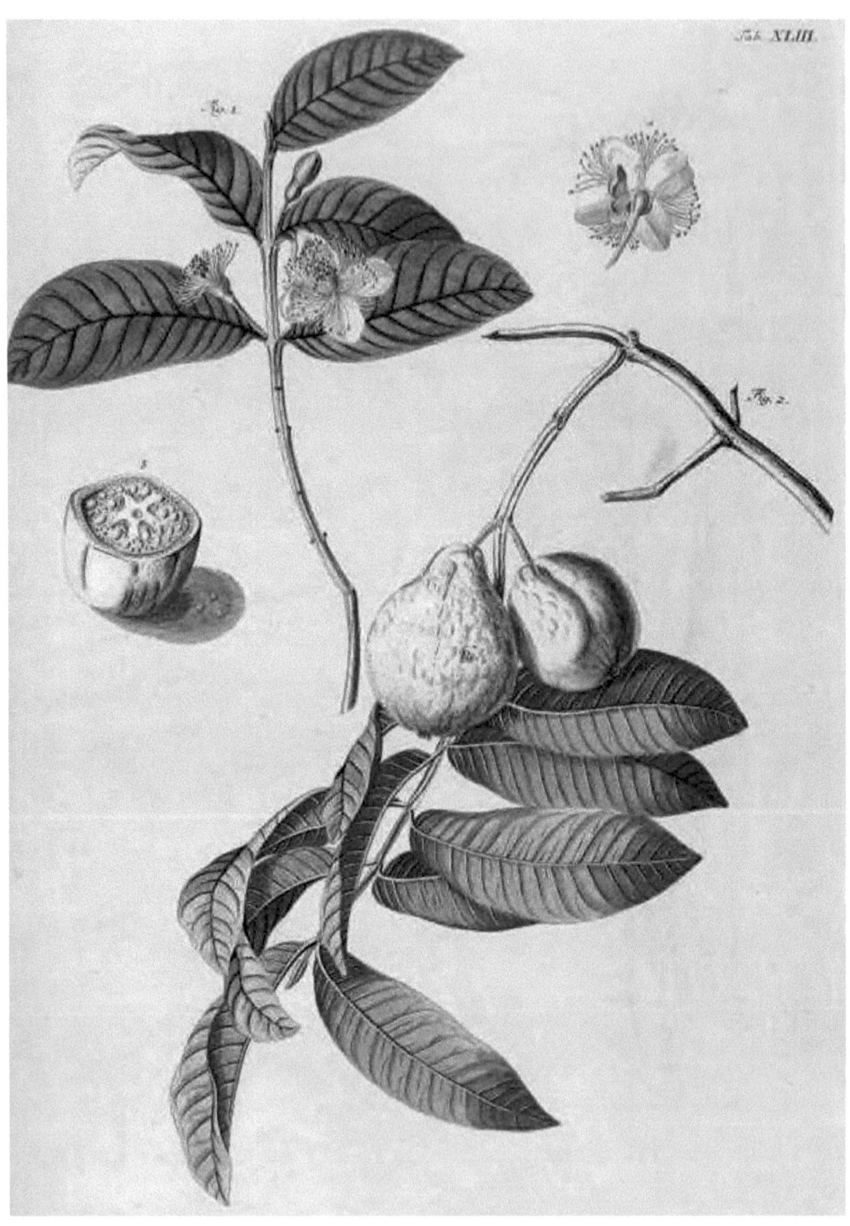

Figura 17. Anatomical illustration of *Psidium guajava* L., from the Myrtaceae family (TREW & EHRET, 1755), which showed activity against *S. schenckii*.

4.5. Plants of the Fabaceae Family

In the Fabaceae family, there are approximately 730 genera covering around 19400 plant species, making it one of the largest botanical families with a wide geographical distribution and which has attracted attention due to its antifungal activities.

Of the few studies on *Sporothrix* spp. in this botanical family, ethyl acetate and ethanolic extracts of the roots of *Glycyrrhiza glabra* from India inhibited isolates with diameters between 7 and 5 mm. This plant is known in Brazil as regaliz or licorice. This plant has sweet roots that are rich in the chemical compound called glabridin (Figure 18), which showed antifungal activity against *S. schenckii* at an inhibition zone of 6 mm. The antifungal activity of glabridin seems to be related to the damage caused to the fungal cell, reducing its cell size and increasing the permeability of the membrane, thus promoting the fungistatic effect. Glabridin is an isoflavone from the flavonoid class and is found in high concentrations in the roots of the *Glycyrrhiza glabra* plant (Figure 19).

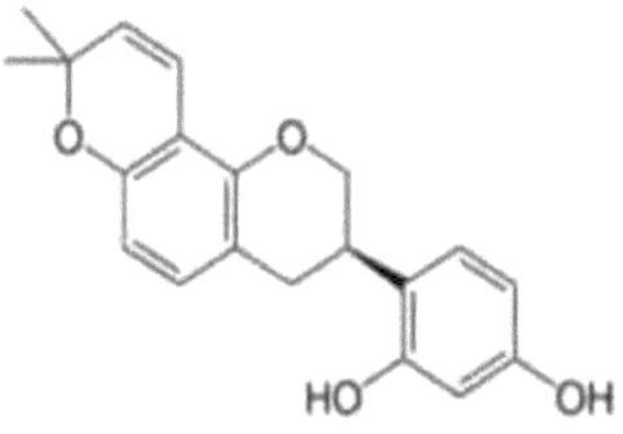

glabridina
($C_{20}H_{20}O_4$)

Figura 18. Chemical structural representation of glabridin, an isoflavone found in the roots of *Glycyrrhiza glabra* with activity against *S. schenckii*.

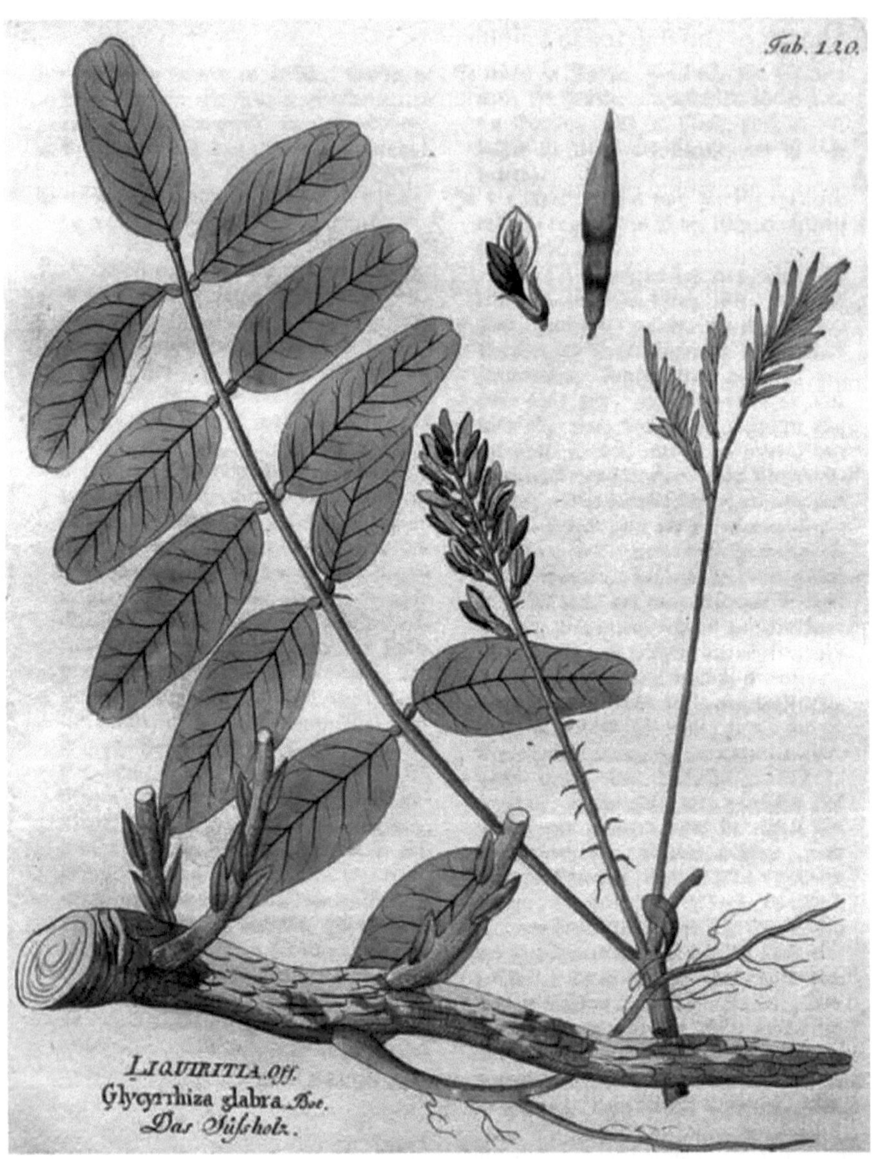

Figura 19. Anatomical illustration of *Glycyrrhiza glabra* L., from the Fabaceae family (VIETZ, 1804), which showed activity against *S. schenckii*.

The *Diphysa robinioides* plant is a shrub that grows between 4 and 15 meters high and is distributed between Mexico and Panama. The ethanolic extract of its leaves inhibited *S. schenckii* in the filamentous phase at a concentration of

1 mg/mL, but this same concentration did not inhibit the yeast phase of the agent.

However, the antifungal activity of the extract at higher concentrations may be present for the yeast phase of the agent, which is the pathogenic phase, and studies should be carried out for this purpose.

Within the Fabaceae family, there is a scientific classification into the subfamily Caesalpiniaseae/Caesalpinioideae, which consists of around 152 genera and around 2700 species distributed in tropical and subtropical regions.

In this subfamily, *Senna alata* (Figure 20) is notable for its medicinal properties. Originally from Mexico, *Senna alata* is known in the region as the "tinea bush", due to its antifungal properties against dermatophytosis and also against malassezia in humans. Ethanolic extracts of the leaves of this plant inhibited the yeast phase of *S. schenckii* at 1 mg/mL.

In the same subfamily, the ethanolic extract of the leaves of *Hymenaea courbaril*, a tree known as jatobà or jatai, was tested at 0.5 mg/mL and inhibited *S. schenckii* in the filamentous phase.

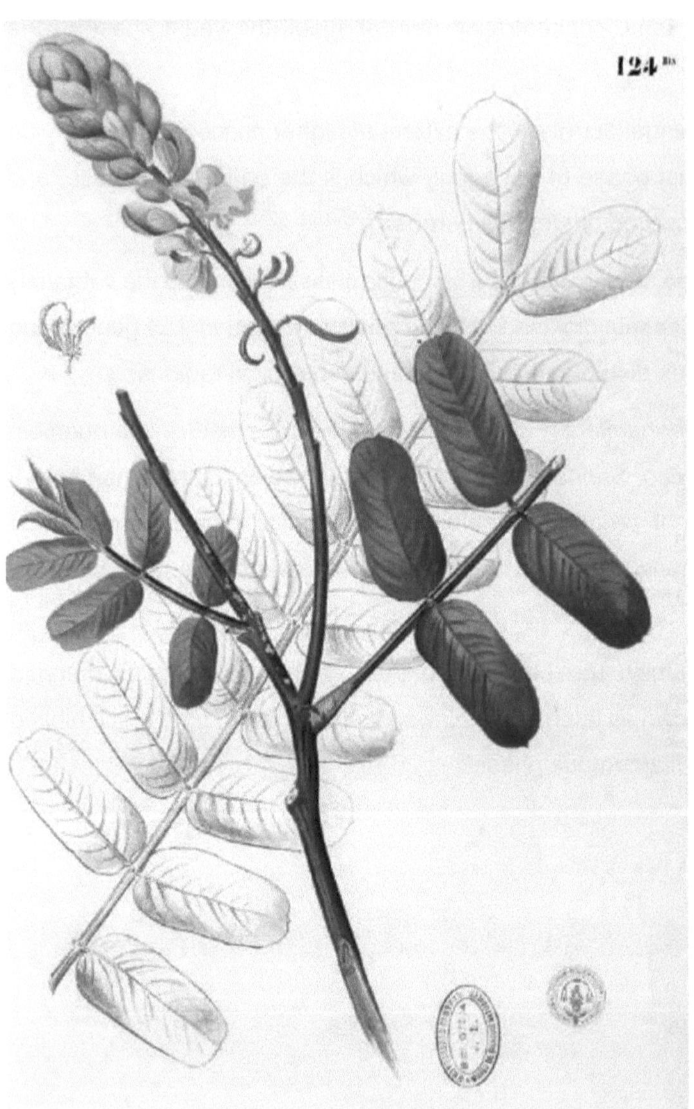

Figura 20. Anatomical illustration of *Senna alata,* from the Fabaceae family (VIETZ, 1804), which showed activity against *S. schenckii*.

4.6. Plants of the Anacardiaceae Family

Represented by around 70 genera containing some 700 species, the Anacardiaceae family is known for its fruit-bearing plants. Among them, is

Schinus terebinthifolius, a tree native to South America, known as red aroeira, which is used in the form of a decoction of the bark to treat inflammation of the cervix and chronic vaginitis, including those of an infectious origin. On *S. schenckii*, extracts of the leaves or stems *of S. terebinthifolius* showed a variation in MIC when prepared in different solvents. The hexanic extracts of the stems and ethanolic extracts of the leaves showed potential, as they were active at a MIC of 15 µg/mL for both types of extractions. The dichloromethane extract of the leaves and ethanolic extract of the stems inhibited at an MIC of 30 µg/mL, while the ethyl acetate extract of the stem was active at an MIC of 60 µg^L.

In plants native to South Africa, Nigeria, Swaziland and other countries, the leaves of the *Protorhus longifolia* (Figure 21) and *Loxostylis alata* trees are popularly used to treat diarrhea and stimulate the immune system, respectively. The hexanic, acetonic, dichloromethane and methanolic extracts of these plants inhibited the growth of *S. schenckii* in 48 hours of observation at MICs between 0.08 and 2.5 mg/mL for *L. alata* and between 0.84 and 2.5 mg/L for *P. longifolia*. Other pathogenic fungi of veterinary importance were also sensitive to the extracts, such as *A. fumigatus, C. albicans, Cryptococcus neoformans* and *M. canis*. In acetone extracts of *Loxostylis alata* leaves, the carbon tetrachloride and butanol fractions were active against *S. schenckii*, at MICs of 0.2 mg/mL and 0.47 mg/mL, respectively, as were the chloroform (0.63 mg/mL), hexane and aqueous methanol (0.71 mg/mL for both) and water (1.88 mg/mL) fractions.

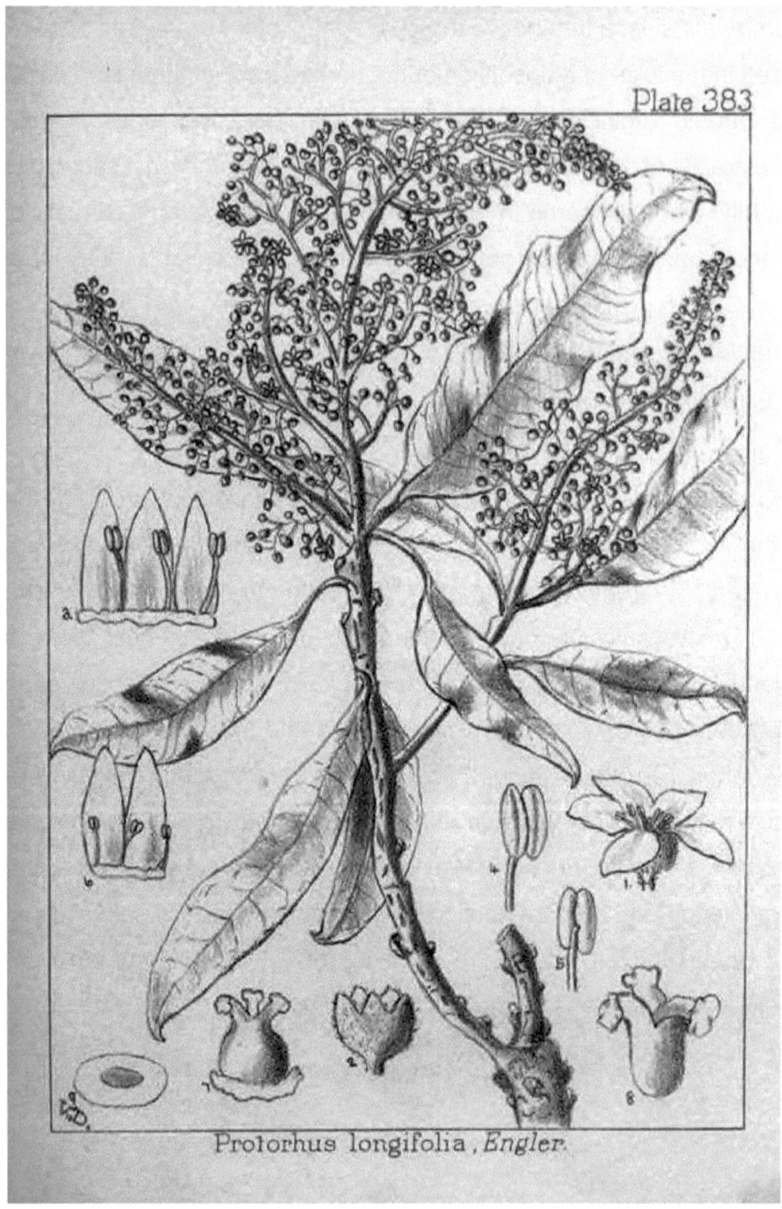

Figure 21. Anatomical illustration of *Protorhus longifolia E.,* from the Anacardiaceae family (WOODS & EVANS, 1903), which showed inhibitory activity against *S. schenckii*.

Agavaceae is a botanical family made up of 24 genera containing around 630 plant species. Originating in North and Central America, mainly in Mexico, plants of the genus *Agave,* such as *A. americana* (Figure 22), are known for storing water in greater quantities than normal plants, as a way of adapting to dry and arid environments, and are called "succulent plants".

The sap of *Agave* spp. is used in folk medicine for its anti-inflammatory, antiseptic, diuretic and laxative properties, as well as stimulating the healing process. These plants are rich in isoflavonoids, alkaloids, coumarins and other chemical compounds. Their soothing properties protect mucous membranes and stimulate healing.

In addition, these plants are recognized for their antimicrobial properties against bacterial and fungal pathogens such as *Cryptococcus neoformans, dermatophytes Microsporum gypseum* and *Trichophyton tonsurans*.

The anti-Sporothrix *schenckii* activity of *Agave* spp. leaves has been demonstrated on clinical isolates of human sporotrichosis. The ethanolic extracts of the leaves of *A. scabra*, *A. lechuguilla, A. lophanta*, and *A. picta* are considered promising, as they show antifungal activity against *S. schenckii*, inhibiting growth in a zone of 9 mm to 16 mm.

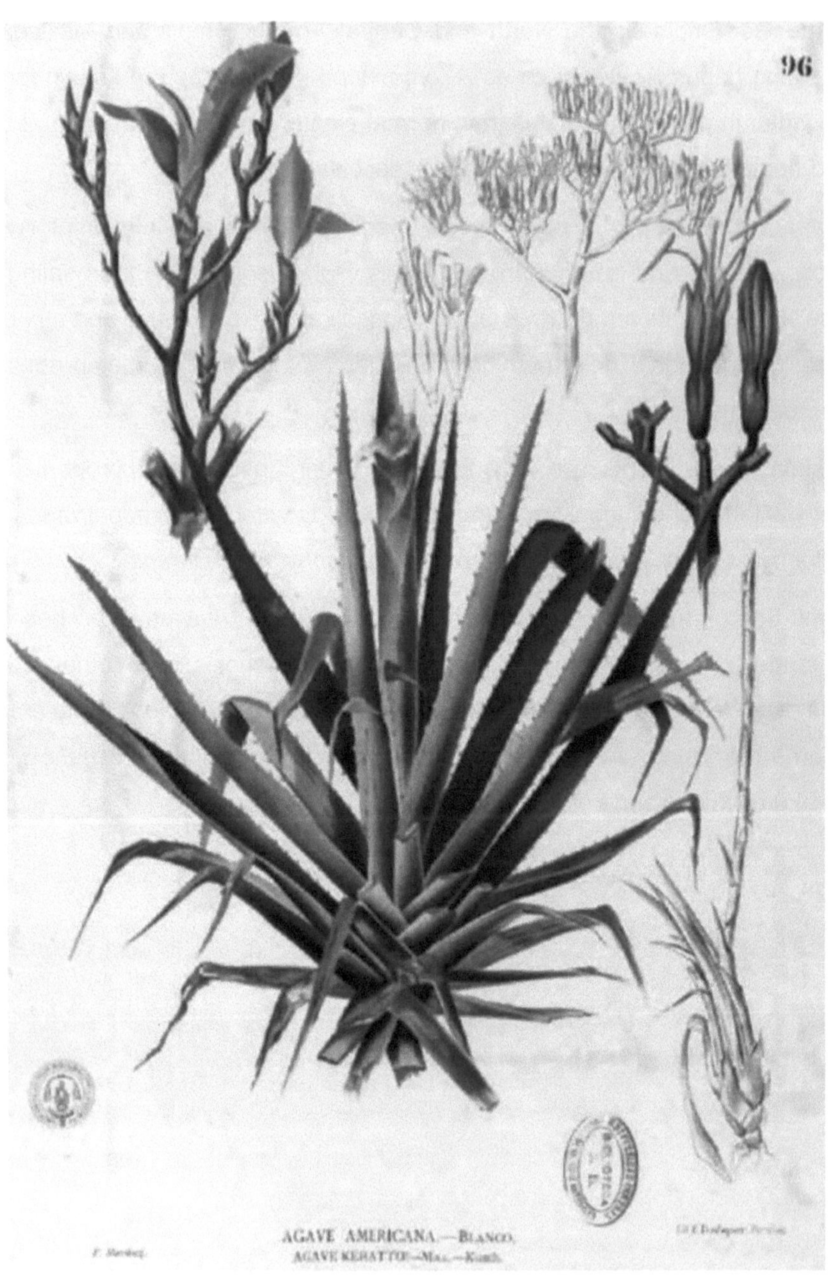

Figure 22. Anatomical illustration of *Agave americana,* from the Agavaceae family (BLANCO, 1875).

4.8. Plants of the Polygalaceae Family

The Polygalaceae family contains around 600 plant species, most of which belong to the *Polygala* genus. Several pharmacological properties have been attributed to *Polygala* species, including antifungal properties against *Cryptococcus gatii* and *Candida* .

Of the active chemical compounds isolated from the *Polygala* sp. plant, α-spinasterol and "1,2,3,4,5,6-hexanehexol" isolated from *P. sabulosa* were active against *S. schenckii* at a MIC of 250 μg/mL, as was "7-methoxy-5-phenyloxycoumarin" at a MIC of 125 μg/mL. The compound α-spinasterol was also isolated from *P. paniculata* and, when tested against *S. schenckii*, it also inhibited it at the MIC of 250 μg^L (Figure 23). In ethanolic extracts of *P. paniculata* (Figure 24) collected in southern Brazil, clinical isolates of *S. schenckii* were sensitive at a MIC of 1000 μg^L. Acetyl-acetate, dichloromethanolic and ethanolic extracts of *P. sabulosa* at a MIC of 30 μgλmL, 250 μg^L and 1000 μgλmL, respectively, and a dichloromethanolic extract of *P. campestris* inhibited the isolates at a MIC of 500 μg^L.

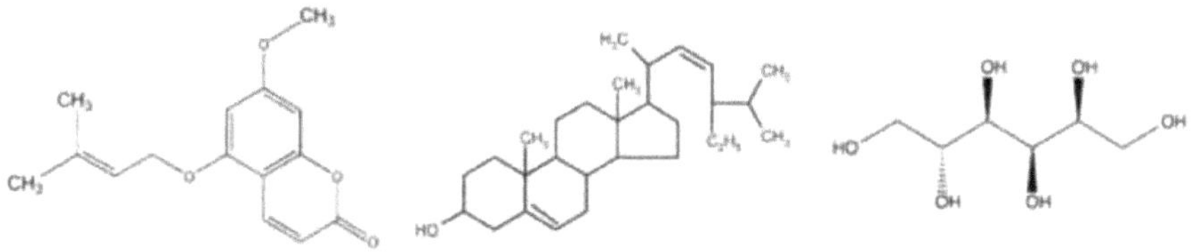

7-metoxi-5-feniloxicumarina ($C_{15}H_{16}O_4$) | α-spinasterol ($C_{29}H_{48}O$) | 1,2,3,4,5,6-hexanehexol ($C_6H_{14}O_6$)

Figure 23. Chemical structural representation of the compounds active against *S. schenckii* and isolated from the plants *Polygala sabulosa* and *Polygala paniculata*, and their respective structural formulas, which showed potential activity against *S. schenckii*.

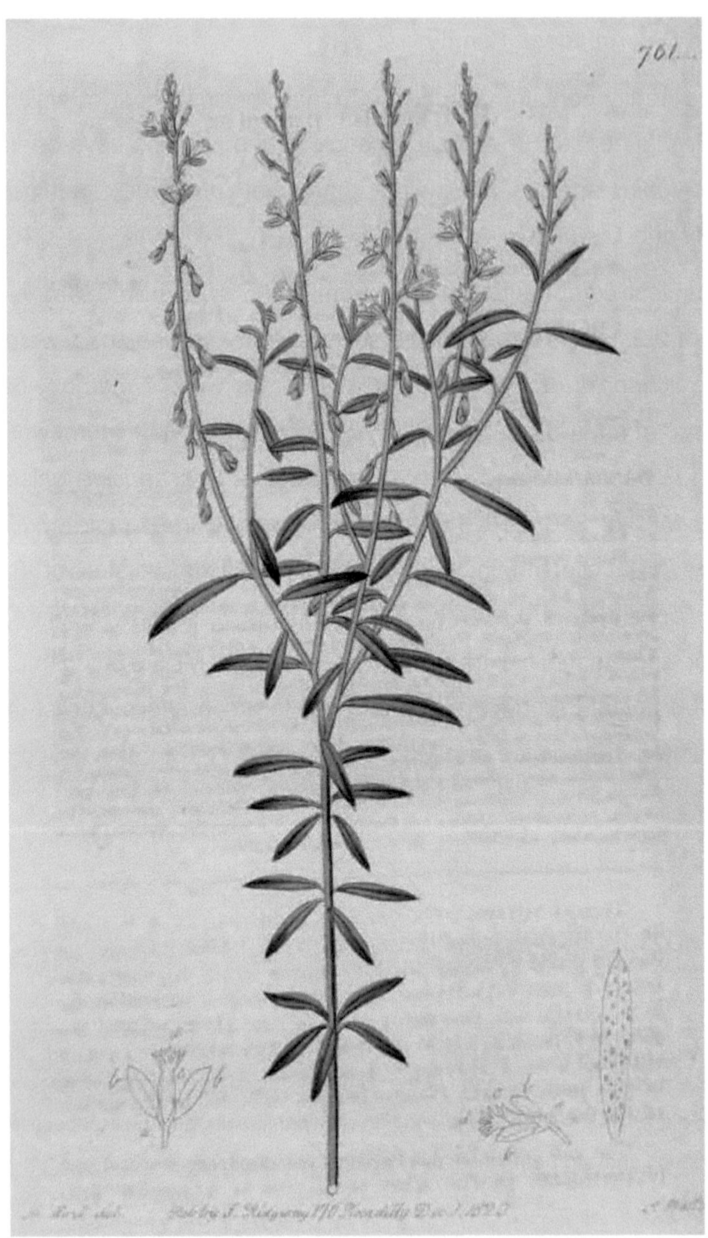

Figure 24. Anatomical illustration of *Polygala paniculata,* from the Polygalaceae family (HART, 1823).

4.8. Plants of the Poaceae Family

In this family are plants of the *Cymbopogon* spp. genus, such as citronella (*C. winterianus*), palmarosa (*C. martinii*) and lemongrass (*C. flexuosus*), which are widely used as insect repellents and showed antimicrobial activity, including antifungal activity. The oils from these plants showed inhibitory potential on the growth of *S. schenckii*, which was inhibited from growing to a zone of 12 and 19 mm for citronella (*C. winterianus*) and palmarosa (*C. martini*), respectively, and up to 35 mm for lemongrass (*C. flexuosus*), which stood out as fungistatic.

Of the chemical compounds active in *Cymbopogon* spp. plants, geraniol, citronellol, citral and citronellal (Figure 25) stand out for their anti-Sporothrix *schenckii* activity. Among the products tested, geraniol showed the best inhibitory potential, as it inhibited the growth of *S. schenckii* when diluted up to 3200x, while lemongrass oil showed the best fungicidal activity, as it caused fungal death when diluted up to 1600x. Lemongrass oil enriched with geraniol seems to be a good approach for controlling sporotrichosis.

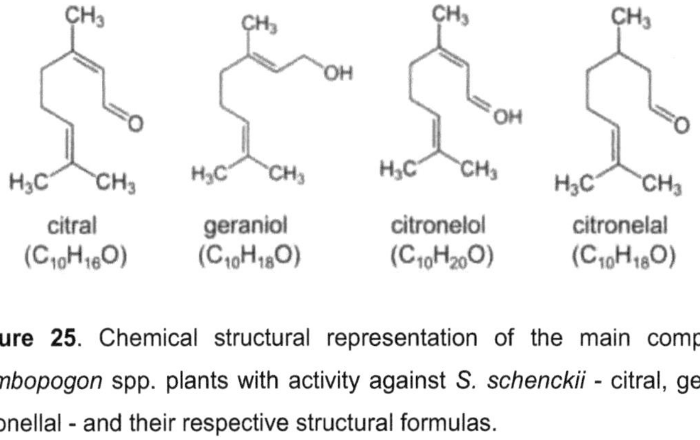

citral ($C_{10}H_{16}O$) | geraniol ($C_{10}H_{18}O$) | citronelol ($C_{10}H_{20}O$) | citronelal ($C_{10}H_{18}O$)

Figure 25. Chemical structural representation of the main compounds identified in *Cymbopogon* spp. plants with activity against *S. schenckii* - citral, geraniol, citroneol and citronellal - and their respective structural formulas.

4.9. Other Botanical Species

Other species from different botanical families have also been researched and have shown antifungal potential against agents of the *Sporothrix schenckii* complex (Table 6), such as green tea, cinnamon, cumin, sorrel, blackberry, among others.

Table 6. Botanical species from different families with proven antifungal activity against fungi of the *Sporothrix schenckii* complex and their respective information about the anatomical parts and types of extracts tested.

Species (Family)	**Anatomical part and types of active extracts***
Camellia sinensis (Theaceae)[f]	Aerial parts (Aq)
Cinnamomum zeylanicum (Lauraceae) [c]	Cortex (He)
Cuminum cyminum (Apiaceae)[a]	Seed (Aq, EO, Ha, M)
Curtisia dentata (Cornaceae)[b]	Leaves, Stems (Ac, Di, He, M)
Lippia graveolens (Verbenaceae)[g,h]	Leaves (E, He)
Piper abutiloides (Piperaceae)[d]	Aerial Parts (Ha)
Rubus urticaefolius (Rosaceae)[e]	Leaves, Stems, Flowers (E, EA)
Rumex acetosa (Polygonaceae)[e]	Leaves, Stems, Flowers (E)
Smilax domingensis (Smilacaceae)[g]	Leaves, Stems, Roots, Flowers (E)
Valeriana prionophylla (Valerianaceae)[g]	Roots (E)

[a] Chaudhary *et al.*, 2014; [b] Shai *et al.*, 2008; [c] Màrquez, 2010; [d] Johann *et al.*, 2009; [e] Johann *et al.*, 2007; [f] Waller *et al.*, 2015; [g] Fernândez, 2005; [h] Beteta, 2006;

[a] Chaudhary *et al.*, 2014; [b] Shai *et al.*, 2008; [c] Márquez, 2010; [d] Johann *et al.*, 2009; [e] Johann *et al.*, 2007; [f] Waller *et al.*, 2015; [g] Fernández, 2005; [h] Beteta, 2006; * Ac - acetone; Aq - aqueous; Di - dichloromethane; E - ethanol; EA - ethyl acetate; Há - hydroalcoholic; He - hexane; OE - essential oil; M - methanol.

In the Theaceae family, the *Camellia sinensis* plant *is* popularly consumed as tea, and its varieties are known as green tea, black tea, white tea, Oolong tea, among others. In *the case of S. brasiliensis* isolated from dogs and cats with sporotrichosis and *S. schenckii* isolated from humans, inhibitory activity was observed in green tea prepared as an infusion and decoction, with MIC values ranging from$\leq$ 1.56 to 6.25 mg/ml. The antifungal potential of this plant is also recognized by its inhibitory activity on clinical isolates resistant to itraconazole.

In the Lauraceae family, the *Cinnamomum zeylanicum* plant is widely used in cooking and perfumery in many countries around the world and is popularly known as cinnamon. Studies into its antifungal potential have been promising.

In Mexico, the hexanic extract from the plant's cortex inhibited the growth of *S. schenckii* by 14 mm.

In the Apiaceae family, the antimicrobial activity of the seeds of *Cuminum cyminum* (Figure 26), native to Egypt and Syria, has already been recognized against various antimicrobial pathogens. This plant is popularly known as cumin, an herb widely used in cooking around the world. Carminative, analgesic, antispasmodic, astringent and eupeptic properties are recognized in cumin seeds, as well as being used to treat digestive disorders such as diarrhea, flatulence and colic, as well as to relieve respiratory symptoms such as coughs and dyspnea, headaches, liver dysfunction, among others.

In India, different extractions of cumin at a concentration of 0.5 mg/mL were active against *S. schenckii*. The essential oil of cumin showed the best activity, producing an inhibition zone of 18 mm, followed by the methanolic extract with 12 mm and the hydroalcoholic extract with 3 mm. The aqueous extract of this plant showed no antifungal activity.

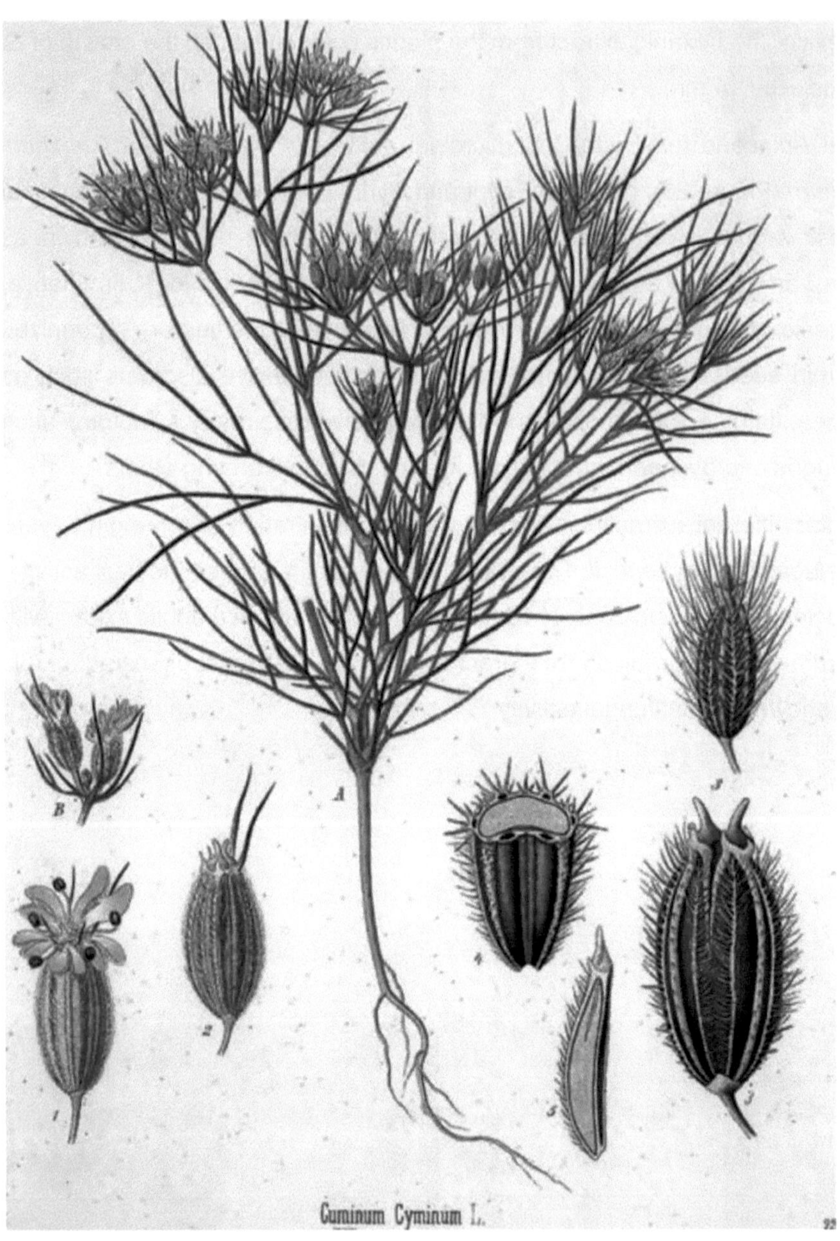

Figura 26. Anatomical illustration of *Cuminum cyminum* L., from the Apiaceae family (KOHLER, 1890).

The antifungal activity of *Cuminum cyminum* was related to the majority composition of the essential oil, especially the compounds trans-dihydrocarvone, γ-terpinene and p-cymene (Figure 27), which already showed antifungal activity when tested alone.

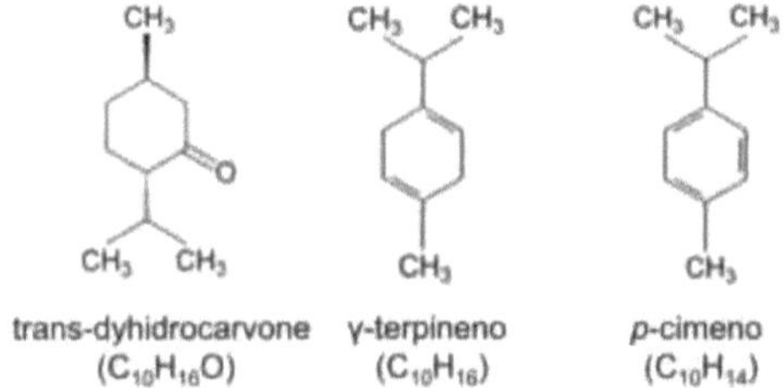

Figura 27. Chemical structural representation of the major compounds identified in the essential oil of *Cuminum cyminum* - trans-dihydrocarvone, γ-terpinene and p-cymene.

In South Africa, *Curtisia dentata* is a tree of the Cornaceae family used to treat bacterial and fungal diseases. Among the active compounds (Figure 28) in the dichloroform extracts of *C. dentata* leaves (Figure 29), lupeol showed the best activity against *S. schenckii* at a MIC of 12 μg/mL, followed by betulinic acid at 16 μg/mL, 2α-hydroxyursOlic acid at 24 μg/mL and ursolic acid at 32 μg/mL.

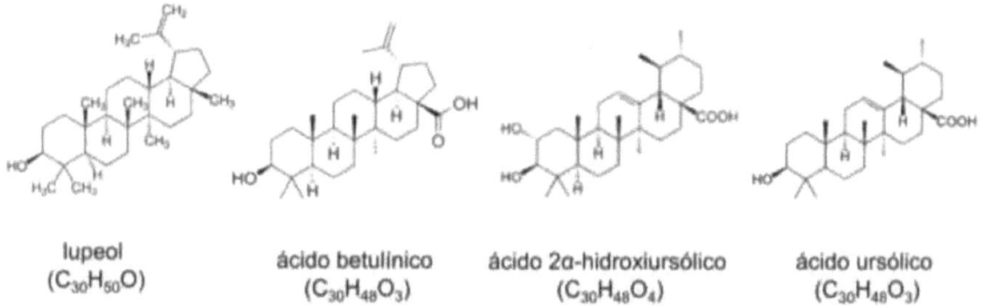

Figure 28. Chemical structural representation of the compounds active against *S. schenckii* identified in the extracts of *Curtisia dentata* leaves - lupeol, betulinic acid, 2α-hydroxyursOlic acid and ursolic acid - in decreasing order of antifungal potential.

Pag. 235.
Tab. LXXXII
SIDEROXYLUM foliis acuminatis, dentatis,
fructu monopyreno, flavo.
b
a

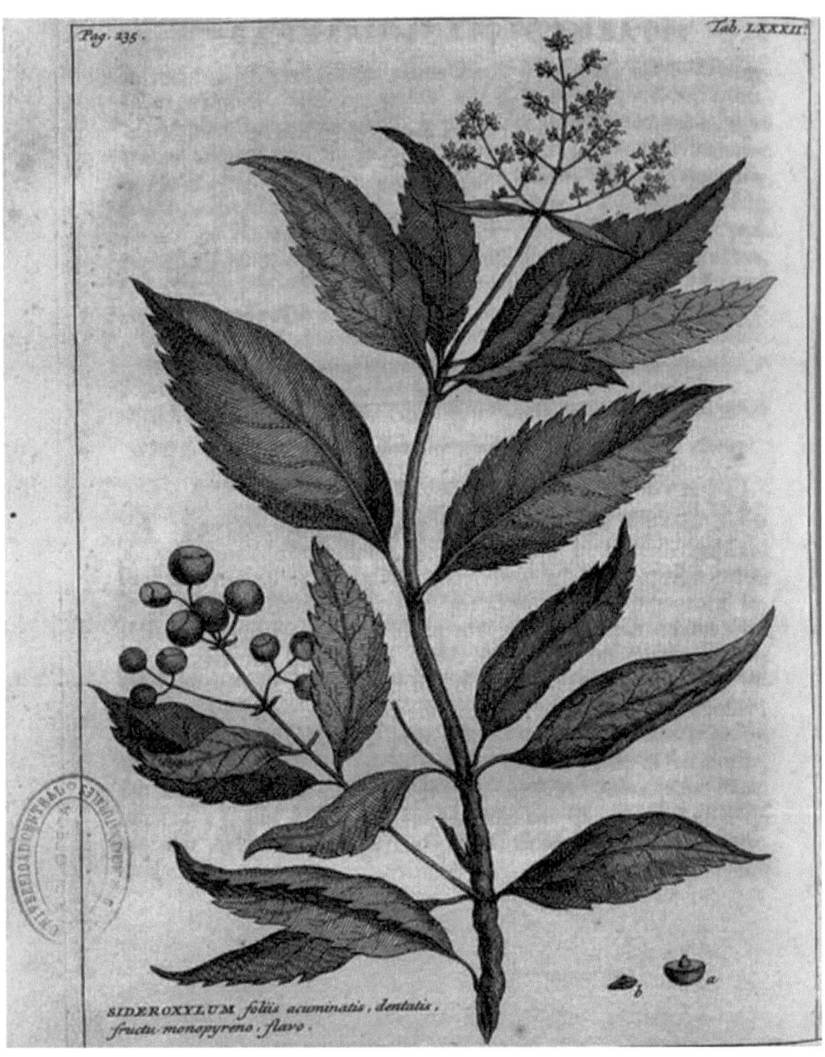

Figure 29. Anatomical illustration of *Curtisia dentata* L., from the Cornaceae family (BURMAN, 1739).

In the Piperaceae family, there are 10 genera with around 200 species with antimicrobial, antiviral, antioxidant and antiparasitic properties, among others. In Brazil, the species *P. abutiloides* has been recognized against *S. schenckii* in the form of a hydroalcoholic extract with a MIC of 125 µg/mL, as well as its isolated compounds, which showed MIC activity of 12.5 µg/mL for pseudillapiol,

25 μg/mL for eupomatenoid-6 and 50 μg/mL for conocarpan (Figure 30).

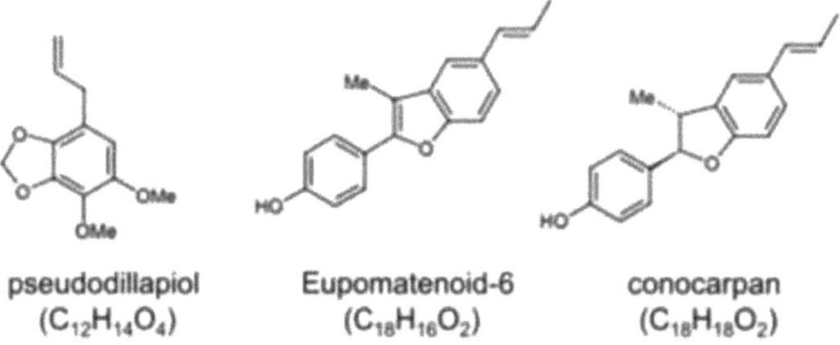

Figure 30. Chemical structural representation of the compounds pseudodillapiol, epomatenoi- 6 and conocarpan, isolated from the hexane fraction of the hydroalcoholic extract of the aerial parts of *Piper abutiloides* and which showed anti-Sporothrix *schenckii* activity when tested alone, and their respective structural formulas.

The antifungal activity of plants collected in southern Brazil has been demonstrated against fungal pathogens, including *S. schenckii*. In the Polygonaceae family, *Rumex acetosa* (Figure 31) is a plant popularly known as azedeira, and showed anti-Sporothrix *schenckii* activity at a MIC of 1000 μg^L when prepared as an ethanolic extract. In the Rosaceae family, the ethanolic and acetyl acetate extracts of *Rubus urticaefolis* were active against *S. schenckii* at a MIC of 125 μg^L. This plant is known in Brazil as blackberry, and is used to treat diarrhea and gastrointestinal disorders, as well as affections of the oral cavity.

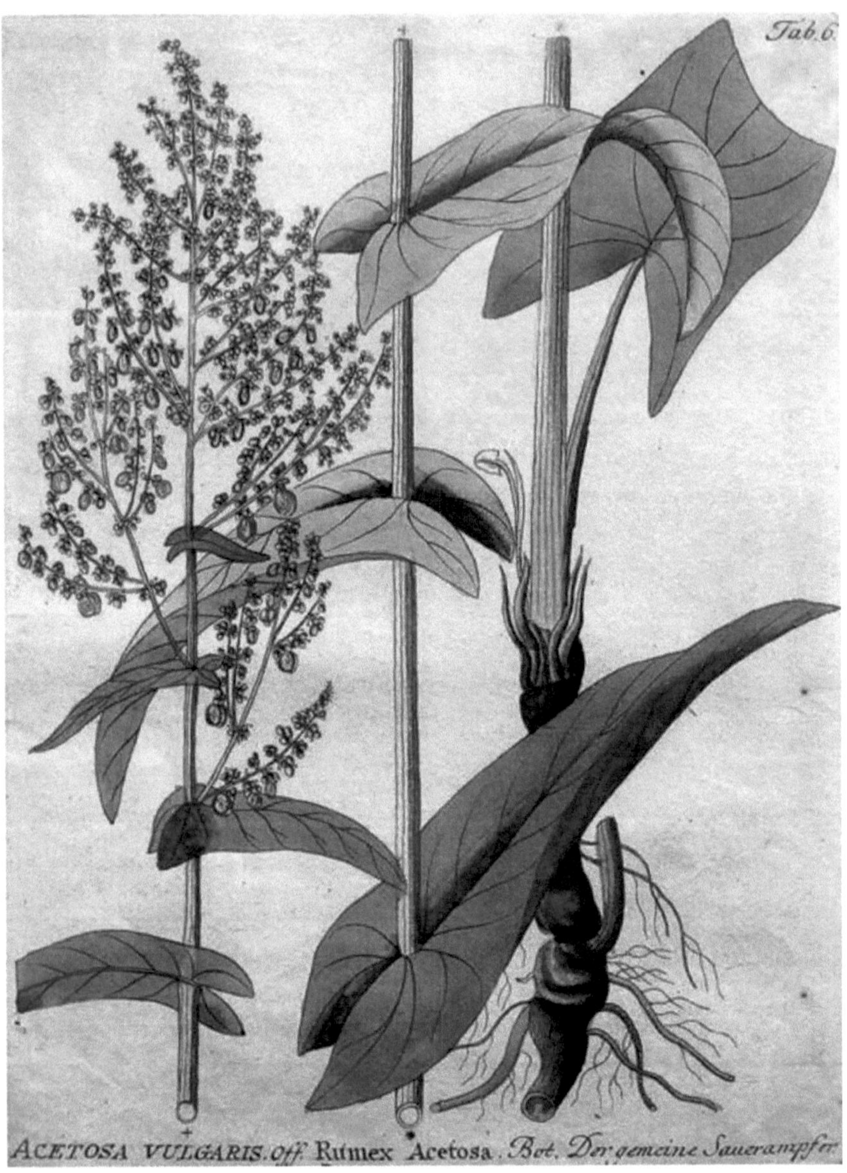

Figure 31. Anatomical illustration of *Rumex acetosa,* from the Polygonaceae family (VIETZ, 1800).

In plants native to Central American countries such as Guatemala, ethanolic extracts of the leaves, stems, flowers and roots of *Smilax domingensis* (family

Smilacaceae) and the roots of *Valeriana prionophylla* (family Valerianaceae) inhibited *S. schenckii at 1 mg/mL. schenckii* at 1 mg/mL, as well as the ethanolic and hexanic extracts of *Lippia graveolens* (family Verbenaceae), which were recognized as promising for the treatment of sporotrichosis, and further studies should be carried out for this purpose.

conclusions

Various therapeutic protocols have been advocated for feline and canine sporotrichosis, mainly through the use of traditional and modern antifungal drugs, and other therapeutic modalities for clinical cases that are refractory to antifungal drugs. Obtaining a clinical cure depends on the sensitivity of the fungal species of the *Sporothrix schenckii* complex, the immune conditions of the animal, as well as the financial and operational willingness of the guardian during therapeutic management. However, the current problem of antifungal resistance has stimulated the search for new active antifungal molecules through medicinal plants. Botanical species from different families have been recognized as having antifungal activity against fungi of the *Sporothrix schenckii* complex in different extractions, and their active molecules have been recognized as antifungal. Further studies should be carried out to assess the safety and efficacy of plant extracts and their molecules in clinical trials. As a future prospect, we believe that new potent drugs can be developed from medicinal plant extracts that can be used to treat sporotrichosis safely and effectively, including in cases that are refractory to antifungal drugs.

COMPLEMENTARY BIBLIOGRAPHY

ADEBOLU, T. T.; OLADIMEJI, S. A. Antimicrobial activity of leaf extracts *of Ocimum gratissimun* on selected diarrhea causing bacteria in SouthWest Nigeria. **African Journal of Biotechnology**, Nairobi, Kenya, v. 4, n. 7, p. 682-684, July, 2005.

AKHTAR, M. M.; SRIVASTAVA, S.; SINHA, P.; SINGH, D.K.; LUQMAN, S.; TANDON, S.; YADAV, N. P. Antimicrobial potential of topical formulation containing essential oil Eucalyptus citriodora Hook. **Annals of Phytomedicine**, Hyderabad, India, v.3, n.1, p.37-42, June, 2014.

ALMEIDA, H. L. JR.; LETTNIN, C. B.; BARBOSA, J. L.; DIAS, M. C. Spontaneous resolution of zoonotic sporotrichosis during pregnancy. **Revista do Instituto de Medicina Tropical de Săo Paulo**, Sâo Paulo, v. 51, n. 4, p. 237-238, July/August, 2009

ALVES, S. H.; BOETTCHER, C.S.; OLIVEIRA, D.C.; TRONCO-ALVES, G.R.; SGARIA, M.A.; THADEU, P.; OLIVEIRA, L.T.; SANTURIO, J.M. *Sporothrix schenckii* associated with armadillo hunting in Southern Brazil: epidemiological and antifungal susceptibility profiles. **Revista da Sociedade Brasileira de Medicina Tropical**, Uberaba, v. 43, n.5, p. 523-525, September/October, 2010.

AMORIM, M.M.R.; SANTOS, L.C. Treatment of bacterial vaginosis with *Schinus terebinthifolius* Raddi vaginal gel: a randomized controlled trial. **Revista Brasileira de Gincecologia e Obstetricia**, Rio de Janeiro, v. 25, n. 2, p. 95-102, March, 2003.

ANTUNES, T. A.; NOBRE, M. O.; FARIA, R. O.; MEINERZ, A. R.; MARTINS, A. A.; CLEFF, M. B.; FERNANDES, C. G.; MEIRELES, M. C. A. Experimental cutaneous sporotrichosis: *in vivo* evaluation of itraconazole and terbinafine. **Revista da Sociedade Brasileira de Medicina Tropical**, Uberaba, v. 42, n.6, p. 706-710, December, 2009.

ARABI, Z.; SARDARI, S. An investigation into the antifungal property of Fabaceae using bioinformatics tools. **Avicenna Journal of Medical Biotechnology**, Tehran, Iran, v.2, n.2, p.93-100, April/June, 2010.

BACKES, L.T.H.; NAUMANN, V.L.D.; CALIL, L.N. Isolation of anemophilic fungi in a library and prevalence of respiratory allergies. **Revista Panamericana de Infectologia**, Sâo Paulo, v.13, n.3, p. 19-25, June, 2011.

BALAKUMAR, S.; RAJAN, S.; THIRUNALASUNDARI, T.; JEEVA, S. Antifungal activity of *Ocimum sanctum* Linn. (Lamiaceae) on clinically isolated dermatophytic fungi. **Asian Pacific of Tropical Medicine**, Haikou, China, v.4, n.8, p.654-657, August, 2011.

BARROS, M. B. L.; PAES, R. A.; SCHUBACH, A. O. *Sporothrix schenckii* and Sporotrichosis. **Clinical Microbiology Reviews**, Washington, United States, v.24, n.4, p.633-654, October, 2011.

BARROS, M.B.L.; SCHUBACH, T.M.P.; COLL, J.O.; GREMIÂO, I.D.; WANKE, B.; SCHUBACH, A. Sporotrichosis: the evolution and challenges of an epidemic. **Revista Panamericana de Salud Pùblica**, Washington, United States, v. 27, n. 6, p.455-460, June, 2010.

BARROS, M.B.L.; SCHUBACH, T.M.P.; GALHARDO, M.C.G.; SCHUBACH, A.O.; MONTEIRO, P.C.F.; REIS, R.S.; ZANCOPÉ-OLIVEIRA, R.M.; LAZÉRA, M.S.; CUZZI-MAYA, T.; BLANCO, T.C.M.; MARZOCHI, K.B.F.; WANKE, B.; VALLE, A.C.F. Sporotrichosis: an emergent zoonosis in Rio de Janeiro. **Memórias do Instituto Oswaldo Cruz**, Rio de Janeiro, v. 96, n.6, p.777-779, August, 2001.

BERNSTEIN, J. A.; COOK, H. E.; GILL, A. F.; RYAN, K.A.; SIRNINGER, J. Cytologic diagnosis of generalized cutaneous sporotrichosis in a hunting hound. **Veterinary Clinical Pathology**, Malden, United States, v. 36, n. 1, p.94-96, March, 2007.

BETETA, Gaudi Haydee Ortiz. **Antifungal Activity of the Extracts**

Ethanolicos de la Flor de *Bourreria huanita* y la Hoja de *Lippia graveolens* y sus Particiones Hexanica, Cloroformica, Acetato de Etilo y Acuosa contra los Hongos *Sporothrix schenckii* y *Fonsecaea pedrosoi*. 69 f. Tesis (Doctorate) - Faculty of Chemical Sciences and Pharmacy, University of San Carlos de Guatemala, Guatemala City, 2005.

BLANCO, M. **Flora de Filipinas** (1875). Available at: http://plantillustrations.org/illustration.php2id illustration=62385. Accessed on: 05 April 2017.

BORBA-SANTOS, L. P.; RODRIGUES, A. M.; GAGINI, T. B.; FERNANDES, G. F.; CASTRO, R.; CAMARGO, Z. P.; NUCCI, M.; LOPES-BEZERRA, L. M.; ISHIDA, K.; ROZENTAL, S.. Susceptibility of *Sporothrix brasiliensis* isolates to amphotericin B, azoles and terbinafine. **Medical Mycology**, Oxford, England, v. 53, n. 2, p.178-188, 2015.

BORGES, Tatiana Saleme. **Isolation of *Sporothrix schenckii* from the claws of domestic cats (domiciled and kenneled) and those kept in captivity in São Paulo (Brazil).** 69 f. Dissertation (Master's Degree) - Faculty of Veterinary Medicine and Zootechny, University of Sao Paulo, Sao Paulo, SP, 2007.

BOZIN, B.; MIMICA-DUKIN, N.; SAMOJLIK, I.; JOVIN, E. Antimicrobial and antioxidant properties of rosemary and sage (*Rosmarinus officinalis* L. and *Salvia officinalis* L., lamiaceae) essential oils. **Journal of Agricultural and Food Chemistry**, Washington, United States, v.55, n. 19, p.7879-7885, August, 2007.

BRILHANTE, R. S.; RODRIGUES, A. M.; SIDRIM, J. J.; ROCHA, M. F.; PEREIRA, S. A.; GREMIÂO, I. D.; SCHUBACH, T. M.; DE CAMARGO, Z. P. *In vitro* susceptibility of antifungal drugs against *Sporothrix brasiliensis* recovered from cats with sporotrichosis in Brazil. **Medical Mycology**, Oxford, England, v. 54, n. 3, p. 275-279, March, 2016.

BROWN, J.E. **The Forest Flora of South Australia** (1833). Available at: http://plantillustrations.org/illustration.php2id illustration= 96381. Accessed on: 05 April 2017.

BURMAN, J. **Rariorum Africanarum plantarum** (1739). Available at: http://plantillustrations.org/illustration.php2id illustration=234360. Accessed on: April 5, 2017.

CAFARCHIA, C.; SASANELLI, M. T.; LIA, R. P.; CAPRARIIS, D.; GUILLOT, J.; OTRANTO, D. Lymphocutaneous and nasal sporotrichosis in a dog from Southern Italy: Case Report. **Mycopathologia**, The Hague, Netherlands, v.163, n. 2, p.75-79, February, 2007.

CARRADA-BRAVO, T.; OLVERA-MACiAS, M.L. New observations on the ecology and epidemiology of *Sporothrix schenckii* and sporotrichosis. **Revista Latinoamericana de Patologia Clinica y Medicina de Laboratorio**, Mexico, v.60, n. 1, p.5-24, January/March, 2013.

CARVALHO, M.T.M.; CASTRO, A.P.; BABY, C.; WERNER, B.; NETO, J.F.; QUEIROZ-TELLES, F. Disseminated cutaneous sporotrichosis in a patient with AIDS: report of a case. **Revista da Sociedade Brasileira de Medicina Tropical**, Uberaba, v. 35, n. 6, p. 655-659, November/December, 2002.

CASTELLANOS, María José Rivera. **Actividad de Seis Extractos de Hierbas Usadas Medicinalmente Contra Fonsecaea pedrosoi y Sporothrix schenckii**. 49 f. Tesis (Doctorate) - Faculty of Chemical Sciences and Pharmacy - University of San Carlos de Guatemala, Guatemala City, 2007.

CERNICKA, J.; SUBIK, J. Resistance mechanisms in fluconazole-resistant *Candida albicans* isolates from vaginal candidiasis. **International Journal of Antimicrobial Agents**, Amsterdam, Netherlands, v. 27, n. 5, p. 403-408, May, 2006.

CHAN, E. W. C.; KONG, L. Q.; YEE, K. Y.; CHUA, W. Y.; LOO, T. Y. Rosemary and sage outperformed six other culinary herbs in antioxidant and antibacterial properties. **International Journal of Biotechnology for Wellness Industries**, Mississauga, Canada, v.1, n.2, p.142-151,2012.

CHAUDHARY, N.; HUSAIN, S.S.; ALI, M. Chemical composition and antimicrobial activity of volatile oil of the seeds of *Cuminin cyminum* L. **World Journal of Pharmacy and Pharmaceutical Sciences**, Sofia, Bulgaria, v.3, n.7, p.1428-1441, June, 2014.

CHAUMETON, F. P. **Flore médicale - volume 1** (1833). Available at:< http://plantillustrations.org/illustration.php2id_illustration=75624> . Accessed on April 5, 2017.

CHAVAN, P.S.; TUPE, S.G. Antifungal activity and mechanism of action of carvacrol and thymol against vineyard and wine spoilage yeasts. **Food Control**, Kidlington, England, v.46, p.115-120, December, 2014.

CHAVES, A. R., DE CAMPOS, M.P.; BARROS, M.B., DO CARMO, C. N.; GREMIÂO, I. D.; PEREIRA, S. A.; SCHUBACH, T. M. Treatment Abandonment in Feline Sporotrichosis - Study of 147 Cases. **Zoonoses and Public Health**, Berlin, Germany, v. 60, n. 2, p. 149-153, March, 2013.

CLEFF, M.B.; MADRID, I.; MEINERZ, A.R.; MEIRELES, M.C.A. MELLO, J.R.B.; RODRIGUES, M.R.; ESCARENO, J.H. Essential oils against *Candida* spp: *in vitro* antifungal activity of *Origanum vulgare*. **African Journal of Microbiology Research**, Lagos, Nigeria, v. 7, n. 20, p. 2245-2250, May, 2013.

CLEFF, M.B.; MEINERZ, A.M.; SCHUCH, L.F.D.; RODRIGUES, M.R.A.; MEIRELES, M.C.A.; MELLO, J.R.B. *In vitro* activity of *Origanum vulgare* essential oil against *Sporothrix schenckii*. **Arquivo Brasileiro de Medicina Veterinària e Zootecnia**, Belo Horizonte, v. 60, n. 2, p. 513-516, April, 2008.

CLEFF, M.B.; MEINERZ, A.R.; FARIA, R.O.; XAVIER, M.O.; SANTIN, R.; NASCENTE, P.S.; RODRIGUES, M.R.; MEIRELES, M.C.A. Inhibitory activity of oregano essential oil on fungi of medical and veterinary importance. **Arquivo Brasileiro de Medicina Veterinària e Zootecnia**, Belo Horizonte, v. 62, n. 5, p.1291-1294, October, 2010.

CLEFF, M.B.; MEINERZ, A.R.; XAVIER, M.; SCHUCH, L.F.; MEIRELES, M.C.A.; RODRIGUES, M.R.A.; MELLO, J.R.B. *In vitro* activity of *Origanum vulgare* essential oil against *Candida* species. **Brazilian Journal of Microbiology**, Sao Paulo, v. 41, n. 1, p. 116-123, January/March, 2010.

CLEFF, M.B.; MEINERZ, A.R.M.; MADRID, I., FONSECA, A. O.; ALVES, H. H.; MEIRELES, M. C. A.; RODRIGUES, M. R. A. Susceptibility profile of yeasts of the genus *Candida* isolated from animals to the essential oil of *Rosmarinus officinalis* L. **Revista Brasileira de Plantas Medicinais**, Botucatu, v.14, n. 1, p.43-49, 2012.

COLODEL, M. M.; JARK, P. C.; RAMOS, C. J. R.; MARTINS, V. M. V.; SCHNEIDER, A. F.; PILATI, C. Feline cutaneous sporotrichosis in the state of Santa Catarina: case report. **Veterinària em Foco**, Canoas, v.7, n.1, p. 18-27, July/December, 2009.

CONTI-DiAZ, I.A., CIVILA, E.; GEZUELE, E.; LOWINGER, M.; CALEGARI, L.; SANABRIA, D.; FUENTES, L.; DA ROSA, D.; ALZUETA, G. Treatment of human cutaneous sporotrichosis with itraconazole. **Mycoses**, Berlin, Germany, v.35, n. 5-6, p.153-156, May/June, 1992.

CORGOZINHO, K.B.; SOUZA, H.J.M.; NEVES, A.; FUSCO, M.A.; BELCHIOR, C. An atypical case of feline sporotrichosis. **Acta Scientiae Veterinariae**, Porto Alegre, v. 34, n. 2, p. 167-170, Februrary, 2006.

CORTÉS, J. A.; RUSSI, J. A. Echinocandins. **Revista Chilena de Infectologia**, Santiago, Chile, v. 28, n. 6, p. 529-536, December, 2011.

COSKUN, B.; SARAL, Y.; AKPOLAT, N.; ATASEVEN, A.; ÇIÇEK, D. Sporotrichosis successfully treated with terbinafine and potassium iodide: case report and review of the literature. **Mycopathologia**, The Hague, Netherlands, v. 158, n. 1, p. 53-56, July, 2004.

COUTO, C.S.F.; RAPOSO, N.R.B.; ROZENTAL, S.; BORBA-SANTOS, L.P.;

BEZERRA, L.M.L.; ALMEIDA, P.A.; BRANDÂO, M.A.F. Chemical composition and antifungal properties of essential oil of *Origanum vulgare* Linnaeus (Lamiaceae) against *Sporothrix schenckii* and *Sporothrix brasiliensis*. **Tropical Journal of Pharmaceutical Research**, Benin city, Nigeria, v. 14, n. 7, p. 1207-1212, July, 2015.

CRISEO, G.; MALARA, G.; ROMEO, O.; PUGLISI GUERRA, A. Lymphocutaneous sporotrichosis in an immunocompetent patient: a case report from extreme southern Italy. **Mycopathologia**, The Hague, Netherlands, v. 166, n. 3, p. 159-162, September, 2008.

CROCE, J.; SILVA, E.G.M.; FURTADO, E.L.; QUELUZ, T.H.A.T. Estudo dos fungos anemófilos da cidade de Botucatu e sua correlação com sensibilização em pacientes com doenças alérgicas respiratórias. **Revista Brasileira de Alergia e Imunopatologia**, Sâo Paulo, v. 26, n. 3, p. 95-109, 2003.

CROTHERS S. L.; WHITE S. D.; IHRKE O. J.; AFFOLTERT V. K. Sporotrichosis: a retrospective evaluation of 23 cases seen in northern California (1987-2007). **Veterinary Dermatology**, Oxford, England, v. 20, n. 4, p. 249-259, August, 2009.

CRUZ, L.C.H. *Sporothrix schenckii* complex. Review of the literature and considerations on diagnosis and epidemiology. **Veterinària e Zootecnia**, Sâo Paulo, v.20, p.8-28, 2011.

DA ROSA, A.C.; SCROFERNEKER, M.L.; VETTORATO, R.; GERVINI, R.L.; VETTORATO, G.; WEBER, A. Epidemiology of sporotrichosis: a study of 304 cases in Brazil. **Journal of the American Academy of Dermatology**, St. Louis, United States, v.52, n. 3, p.451-459, March, 2005.

DABOIT, T.C.; STOPIGLIA, C.D.O.; VON POSER, G.; SCROFERNEKER, M.L. Antifungal activity of *Pterocaulon alopecuroides* (Asteraceae) against chromoblastomycosis agents. **Mycoses**, Berlin, Germany, v. 53, n. 3, p.246-250, May, 2010.

DAFERERA, D.J.; ZIOGAS, B.N.; POLISIOU, M.G. The effectiveness of plant essential oils in the growth of *Botrytis cinerea*, *Fusarium* sp. and *Clavibacter michiganensis* subsp. *michiganensis*. **Crop Protection**, Guildford, England, v. 22, n. 1, p. 39-44, February, 2003.

DAMIALIS, A.; MOHAMMAD, A.B.; HALLEY, J.M.; GANGE, A.C. Fungi in a changing world: growth rates will be elevated, but spores production may decrease in future climates. **International Journal of Biometeorology**, New York, United States, v. 59, n. 9, p. 1157-1167, September, 2015.

DAMIAN-BADILLO, L.M.; SALGADO-GARCIGLIA, R.; MARTiNEZ-MUNOZ, R.E.; MARTiNEZ-PACHECO, M.M. Antifungal properties of some Mexican medicinal plants. **The Open Natural Products Journal**, Sharjah, United Arab Emirates, v.1, n. 1, p.27-33, September, 2008.

DAMODARAN, S.; VENKATARAMAN, S. A study on the therapeutic efficacy of *Cassia alata*, Linn. leaf extract against Pityriasis versicolor. **Journal of Ethnopharmacology**, Lausanne, Ireland, v.42, n. 1, p. 19-23, March, 1994.

DE ARAUJO, T.; MARQUES, A.C.; KERDEL, F. Sporotrichosis. **International Journal of Dermatology**, Oxford, England, v.40, n. 1, p.737742, December, 2001.

DEWICK, Paul M. **Medicinal Natural Products: a Biosynthetic Approach**. 3rd ed. Chinchester: John Wiley & Sons Ltd, 2011.

DIAS, N.M.; OLIVEIRA, M.M.E.; PORTELA, M.A.; SANTOS, C.; ZANCOPE-OLIVEIRA, R.M.; LIMA, N. Sporotrichosis caused by *Sporothrix mexicana*, Portugal. **Emerging Infectious Diseases**, Atlanta, United States, v. 17, n. 10, p. 1975-1976, October, 2011.

DOHERTY, C. B.; DOHERTY, S. D.; ROSEN, T. Thermotherapy in dermatologic infections, **Journal of the American Academy of Dermatology**, St. Louis, United States, v. 62, n. 6, p. 909-927, June, 2010.

DOLD, A.P.; COCKS, M.L. Traditional veterinary medicine in the Alice district of Eastern Cape Province, South Africa. **South African Journal of Science**, Johannesburg, South Africa, v. 97, p. 375-379, 2001.

EATON, M.E. **Addisonia - volume 16** (1931). Available at: < http://plantillustrations.org/illustration.php2id_illustration=162866> . Accessed on: April 05, 2017.

EBADI, Manuchair. **Pharmacodynamic Basis of Herbal Medicine**. 2nd edition. Taylor & Francis Group: Boca Raton, USA. 2006.

ELLIS, D. Amphotericin B: spectrum and resistance. **Journal of Antimicrobial Chemotherapy**, London, England, v.49, n.S1, p.7-10, February, 2002.

ELOFF, J.N. The antibacterial activity of 27 southern African members of the Combretaceae. **South African Journal of Science**, Johannesburg, South Africa, v. 95, p. 148-152, January, 1999.

FABRI, R.L.; NOGUEIRA, M.S.; DUTRA, L.B.; BOUZADA, M.L.M.; SCIO, E. Antioxidant and antimicrobial potential of species from the Asteraceae family. **Revista Brasileira de Plantas Medicinais**, Botucatu, v.13, n.2, p.183-189, 2011.

FARIA, Renata Osório de. **Evaluation of β-(1-3) glucan therapy associated with fluconazole in experimental cryptococcosis**. UFRGS, 2010. Thesis (Doctorate) - Faculty of Veterinary Medicine, Federal University of Rio Grande do Sul, Porto Alegre, RS, 2010.

FAROOQI, Azhar Ali; SREERAMU, B. S. **Cultivation of medicinal and aromatic crops.** Universities Press: India, 2004.

FATIMA, A.; GUPTA, V.K.; LUQMAN, S.; NEGI, A.S.; KUMAR, J.K.; SHANKER, K.; SAIKIA, D.; SRIVASTAVA, S.; DAROKAR, M.P.; KHANUJA, S.P.S. Antifungal Activity of Glycyrriza glabra Extracts and its Active Constituent Glabridin. **Phytotherapy Research**, London, England, v.23, n.8, p.1190-1193, August, 2009.

FERNANDEZ, Isabel Cristina Gaitàn Fernàndez. **Actividad de Doce Plantas Nativas Guatematecas Contra *Sporothrix schenckii*.** 61 f. Thesis (Doctorate) - Faculty of Chemical Sciences and Pharmacy, University of San Carlos de Guatemala, Ciudad de Guatemala, 2005.

FERNANDEZ-SILVA, F.; CAPILLA, J.; MAYAYO, E.; GUARRO, J. Efficacy of posaconazole in murine experimental sporotrichosis. **Antimicrobial Agents and Chemotherapy**, Washington, United States, v. 56, n. 5, p. 2273-2277, May, 2012.

FERNANDEZ-SILVA, F.; CAPILLA, J.; MAYAYO, E.; GUARRO, J.. Modest efficacy of voriconazole against murine infections by *Sporothrix schenckii* and lack of efficacy against *Sporothrix brasiliensis*. **Mycoses**, Berlin, Germany, v. 57, n. 2, p. 121-124, February, 2014.

FILGUEIRA, K. D. Sporotrichosis in dogs: report of a case in the city of Mossoró, RN. **Ciência Animal Brasileira**, Goiânia, v.10, n.2,

April/June, 2009.

FILIPIN, F.B.; SOUZA, L.C. Therapeutic efficacy of lipid formulations of amphotericin B. **Revista Brasileira de Ciências Farmacêuticas**, Sâo Paulo, v. 42, n. 2, p.167-194, April/June, 2006.

FIUZA, T.S.; SABÓIA-MORAIS, S.M.T.; PAULA, J.R.; TRESVENZOL, L.M.F.; PIMENTA, F.C. Antimicrobial activity of the crude ethanol extract from *Hyptidendron canum* leaves. **Pharmaceutical Biology**, London, England, v. 47, n. 7, p. 640-644, 2009.

FREITAS, J. C. O. C.; MEDEIROS, A. C.; SALES V. S. F. Protection by glucan in an experimental model of sepsis. **Acta Cirûrgica Brasileira**, Sâo Paulo, v.19 n.3, p. 296-307, May/June, 2004.

FREITAS, D.C.; MIGLIANO, M.F., ZANI NETO, L. Sporotrichosis. Observation of a spontaneous case in a domestic cat (*F. catus* L.). **Revista da Faculdade**

de Medicina Veterinària, Sâo Paulo, v. 5, n. 4, p. 601-604, 1956.

FYHRQUIST, P.; MWASUMBI, L.; HAEGGSTROM, C.A.; VUORELA, H.; HILTUNEN, R.; VUORELA, P. Ethnobotanical and antimicrobial investigation of some species of *Terminalia* and *Combretum* (Combretaceae) growing in Tanzania. **Journal of Ethnopharmacology**, Lausanne, Ireland, v. 79, n. 2, p. 169-177, February, 2002.

GAITAN, I.; PAZ, A.M.; ZACCHINO, S.A.; TAMAYO, G.; GIMÉNEZ, A.; PINZÓN, R.; CACERES, A.; GUPTA, M.P. Subcutaneous antifungal screening of Latin America plant extracts against *Sporothrix schenckii* and *Fonsecaea pedrosoi*. **Pharmaceutical Biology**, London, England, v.49, n.9, p.907-919, September, 2011.

GENARO, G. Domestic cat - behavior & veterinary practice. **Revista Cientifica de Medicina Veterinària - Pequenos Animais e Animais de Estimaçâo**, Curitiba, v. 3, n.9, p.16-22, 2005.

GOVENDER, N.P.; MAPHANGA, T.G.; ZULU, T.G.; PATEL, J.; WALAZA, S.; JACOBS, C.; EBONWU, J.I.; NTULI, S.; NAICKER, S.D.; THOMAS, J. An Outbreak of Lymphocutaneous Sporotrichosis among Mine-Workers in South Africa. **PLoS Neglected Tropical Diseases**, San Francisco, United States, v. 25, n. 9, p. e0004096, September, 2015.

GREENE Craig.E. **Infectious diseases of the dog and cat**. 4th ed. Philadelphia: W.B. Saunders Company, 2012.

GREMIÂO, I.D.F.; MIRANDA, L.H.M.; REIS, E.G.; RODRIGUES, A.M.; PEREIRA, S.A. Zoonotic Epidemic of Sporotrichosis: Cat to Human Transmission. **PLoS Pathogens**, San Francisco, United States, v. 13, n.1, p.e1006077, January, 2017.

GREMIÂO, I. D. F.; PEREIRA, A. S.; RODRIGUES, A. M.; FIGUEIREDO, F. B.; NASCIMENTO Jr, A.; SANTOS, I. B.; SCHUBACH, T. M. P. Surgical treatment associated with conventional antifungal therapy in feline sporotrichosis. **Acta Scientae Veterinariae**, Porto Alegre, v. 34, n. 2, p. 221-223, February, 2006.

GREMIÂO, I. D. F.; SCHUBACH, T. M. P.; PEREIRA, A. S.; RODRIGUES, A. M.; CHAVES, A. R.; BARROS, M. B. L. Intralesional amphotericin B in a cat with refractory localized sporotrichosis. **Journal of Feline Medicine and Surgery**, London, England, v. 11, n. 8, p. 720-723, August, 2009.

GREMIÂO, I. D. F.; SCHUBACH, T. M. P.; PEREIRA, A. S.; RODRIGUES, A. M.; HONSE, C. O.; BARROS, M. B. L.. Treatment of refractory feline sporotrichosis with a combination of intralesional amphotericin B and oral itraconazole. **Australian Veterinary Journal**, Victoria, Australia, v. 89, n. 9, p. 346-351, September, 2011.

GUERRA-BOONE, L.; ALVAREZ-ROMAN, R.; SALAZAR-ARANDA, R.; TORRES-CIRIO, A.; RIVAS-GALINDO, V.M.; TORRES, N.W.; GONZALEZ, G.; PÉREZ-LÓPEZ, A. Antimicrobial and antioxidant activities and chemical characterization of essential oils of *Thymus vulgaris*, *Rosmarinus officinalis* and *Origanum majorana* from northeastern México. **Pakistan Journal of Pharmaceutical Sciences**, Karashi, Pakistan, v. 28, n. 1, p. 363-369, January, 2015.

GURCAN, S.; KONUK, E.; KILIÇ, H.; OTKUN, M.; ENER, B. Sporotrichosis, a disease rarely reported from Turkey, and an overview of Turkish literature. **Mycoses**, Berlin, Germany, v. 50, n. 5, p. 426-429, September, 2007.

GUTERRES, K.A.; MATOS, C.B.; OSÓRIO, L.G.; SCHUCH, I.D.; CLEFF, M.B. The use of (1-3) β-glucan along with itraconazole against canine refractory sporotrichosis. **Mycopathologia**, The Hague, Netherlands, v.177, n.3-4, p.217-221, April, 2014.

HAMMER, K.A.; CARSON, C.F.; RILEY, T.V. Antifungal activity of the components of *Melaleuca alternifolia* (tea tree) oil. **Journal of Applied Microbiology**, Oxford, England, v.95, n.4, p.853-860, 2003.

HAN, H.S.; KANO, R.; CHEN, C.; NOLI, C. Comparison of two *in vitro* antifungal sensitivity tests and monitoring during therapy of *Sporothrix schencki* sensu stricto in Malaysian cats. **Veterinary Dermatology**, Oxford, England, v. 28, n. 1, p. 156-e32, February, 2017.

HART, M. **Botanical Register - volume 9** (1823). Available at: http://plantillustrations.org/illustration.php2id illustration=98868. Accessed on: 05 April 2017.

HARVEY, W.H. **Thesaurus capensis, or illustrations of South African flora - volume 1** (1859). Available at: **http://plantillustrations.org/illustration.php2id illustration=28988. Accessed on: 05 April 2017.**

HIRANO, M.; WATANABE, K.; MURAKAMI, M.; KANO, R.; YANAI, T.; YAMAZOE, K., FUKATA, T.; KUDO, T. A case of feline sporotrichosis. **The Journal of Veterinary Medical Science**, Tokyo, Japan, v. 68, n. 3, p. 283284, March, 2006.

HIRUMA, M.; KAGAWA, S. Ultrastructure of *Sporothrix schenckii* treated with iodine-potassium iodide solution. **Mycopathologia**, The Hague, Netherlands, v. 97, n. 2, p. 121-127, February, 1987.

HIRUMA, M.; KATOH, T.; YAMAMOTO, I.; KAGAWA, S. Local hyperthermia in the treatment of sporotrichosis. **Mycoses**, Berlin, Germany, v. 30, n. 7, p. 315-321, July, 1987.

HONSE, C. O.; RODRIGUES, A. M.; GREMIÂO, I. D. F.; PEREIRA, A. S.; SCHUBACH, T. M. Use of local hyperthermia to treat sporotrichosis in a cat. **Veterinary Record**, London, England, v. 166, n. 7, p. 208-209, February, 2010.

IACHINI, R. Sporotrichosis in a domestic cat. **Revista Argentina de Microbiologia**, v. 41, n. 1, p.27, January/March, 2009.

JIANG, Y.; WU, N.; FU, Y.J.; WANG, W.; LUO, M.; ZHAO, C. J.; ZU, Y.G.; LIU,

X.L. Chemical composition and antimicrobial activity of the essential oil of Rosemary. **Environmental Toxicology and Pharmacology**, Amsterdam, Netherlands, v.32, n. 1, p. 63-68, July, 2011.

JOHANN, S.; COTA, B.B.; SOUZA-FAGUNDES, E.M.; PIZZOLATII, M.G.; RESENDE, M.A.; ZANI, C.L. Antifungal activities of compounds isolated from *Piper abutiloides* Kunth. **Mycoses**, Berlin, Germany, v.52, n.6, p.499-506, November, 2009.

JOHANN, S.; MENDES, B.G.; MISSAU, F.C.; RESENDE, M.A.; PIZZOLATTI, M.G. Antifungal activity of five species of Polygala. **Brazilian Journal of Microbiology**, Sao Paulo, v.42, n.3, p.1065-1075, July/September, 2011.

JOHANN, S.; PIZZOLATTI, M.G.; DONNICI, C.L.; RESENDE, M.A. Antifungal propertiers of plants used in Brazilian traditional medicine against clinically relevant fungal pathogens. **Brazilian Journal of Microbiology**, Sao Paulo, v.38, n.4, p.632-637, October/December, 2007.

KANO, R.; OKUBO, M.; SIEW, H.H.; KAMATA, H.; HASEGAWA, A. Molecular typing of *Sporothrix schenckii* isolates from cats in Malaysia. **Mycoses**, Berlin, Germany, v. 58, n. 4, p. 220-224, April, 2015.

KAUFFMAN C. A.; BUSTAMANTE B.; CHAPMAN S. W.; PAPPAS P. G. Clinical practice guidelines for the management of sporotrichosis: 2007 update by the Infectious Diseases Society of America. **Clinical Infectious Diseases**, Chicago, United States, v. 45, n. 10, p.1255-1265, November, 2007.

KOHLER, F.E. **Medizinal Pflanzen - volume 3** (1890). Available at: http://plantillustrations.org/illustration.php2id_illustration=31485. Accessed on April 5, 2017.

KOHLER, L. M.; MONTEIRO, P. C. F.; HAHN, R. C.; HAMDAN, S. *In vitro* susceptibilities of isolates of *Sporothrix schenckii* to itraconazole and terbinafine. **Journal of Clinical Microbiology**, Washington, United States, v. 42, n. 9, p. 4319-4320, September, 2004.

KORDALI, S.; CAKIR, A.; MAVI, A.; KILIC, H.; YILDIRIM, A. Determination of the chemical composition and antioxidant activity of the essential oil of *Artemisia dracunculus* and of the antifungal and antibacterial activities of Turkish *Artemisia absinthium*, *A. dracunculus*, *Artemisia santonicum*, and *Artemisia spicigera* essential oils **Journal of Agricultural and Food Chemistry**, Washington, United States, v. 53, n. 24, p. 9452-9458, November, 2005.

LACAZ, Carlos da Silva; PORTO, Edward; MARTINS, José Eduardo Costa; HEINS-VACCARI, Elisabeth Maria; DE MELO, Natalina Takahashi. **Treatise on medical mycology**. 9ªed. Sarvier: Sâo Paulo, 2002.

LAMBERT, R.J.W.; SKANDAMIS, P.N.; COOTE, P.J. A study of the minimum inhibitory concentration and mode of action of oregano essential oil, thymol and carvacrol. **Journal of Applied Microbiology**, Oxford, England, v.91, n. 1, p.453-462, September, 2001.

LARSSON, C.E. Sporotrichosis. **Brazilian Journal of Veterinary Research and Animal Science**, Sâo Paulo, v. 48, n. 3, p. 250-259, 2011.

LEE, Y.S.; KIM, J.; SHIN, S.C.; LEE, S.G.; PARK, I.K. Antifungal activity of Myrtaceae essential oils and their components against three phytopathogenic fungi. **Flavor and Fragance Journal**, Chichester, England, v. 23, n. 1, p.2328, January, 2008.

LEEJA, L.; THOPPIL, E. Antimicrobial activity of methanol extract of *Origanum majorana* L. (sweet marjoram). **Journal of Environmental Biology**, Muzaffarnagar, India, v. 28, n. 1, p.145-146, January, 2007.

LOPES-BEZERRA, L.M.; SCHUBACH, A.; COSTA, R.O. *Sporothrix schenckii* and sporotrichosis. **Annals of the Brazilian Academy of Sciences**, Rio de Janeiro, v. 78, n. 2, p. 293-308, June, 2006.

LÓPEZ-ROMERO, E.; DEL ROCIO REYES-MONTES, M.; PÉREZ-TORRES, A.; RUIZ-BACA, E.; VILLAGÓMEZ-CASTRO, J.C.; MORA-MONTES, H.M.;

FLORES-CARREÓN, A.; TORIELLO, C. *Sporothrix schenckii* complex and sporotrichosis, an emerging health problem. **Future Microbiology**, London, England, v. 6, n. 1, p.85-102, January, 2011.

LUQMAN, S. ; DWIVEDI, G.R. ; DAROKAR, M.P. ; KALRA, A. ; KHANUJA, S.P.S. Potential of Rosemary Oil to be used in Drug-Resistant Infections. **Alternative Therapies in Health Medicine**, Aliso Viejo, United States, v.13, n.5, p.54-59, September/October, 2007.

LUTZ, A.; SPLENDORE, A. On a mycosis observed in men and rats. **Revista de Medicina de Săo Paulo**, Sâo Paulo, v. 21, p. 433-450. 1907.

MACHADO, D. G., BETTIO, L. E. B., CUNHA, M. P., CAPRA, J. C., DALMARCO, J. B., PIZZOLATTI, M. G., RODRIGUES, A. L. Antidepressant-like effect of the extract of *Rosmarinus officinalis* in mice: Involvement of the monoaminergic system. **Progress in Neuro-Psychopharmacology and Biological Psychiatry**, Oxford, England, v. 33, n. 4, p.642-650, June, 2009

MADRID I.M., MATTEI, A.; MARTINS, A., NOBRE, M.; MEIRELES, M. Feline sporotrichosis in the southern region of Rio Grande do Sul, Brazil: clinical, zoonotic and therapeutic aspects. **Zoonoses and Public Health**, Berlin, Germany, v.57, n.2, p.151-154, March, 2010.

MADRID, I. M.; MATTEI, A. S.; FERNANDES, C. G.; NOBRE, M. O.; MEIRELES, M. C. A. Epidemiological findings and laboratory evaluation of sporotrichosis: a description of 103 cases in cats and dogs in southern Brazil. **Mycopathologia**, Berlin, Germany, v. 173, n. 4, p. 265-273, April, 2012.

MAHAJAN, V.K. Sporotrichosis: an overview and therapeutic options. **Dermatology Research and Practice**, Cairo, Egypt, v. 2014, n. 2014, ID 272376, p. 1-13, 2014.

MAIDA, I.; NOSTRO, A.; PESAVENTO, G.; BARNABEI, M.; CALONICO, C.; PERRIN, E.; CHIELLINI, C.; FONDI, M.; MENGONI, A.; MAGGINI, V.; VANNACCI, A.GALLO, E.; BILIA, A.R.; FLAMINI, G.; GORI, L.; FIRENZUOLI,

F.; FANI, R. Exploring the Anti-Burkholderia *cepacia* complex activity of essential oils: a preliminary analysis. **Evidence-Based Complementary and Alternative Medicine**, v. 2014, n. ID 573518, p.1-10, 2014.

MARIMON, R.; CANO, J.; GENÉ, J.; SUTTON, D. A.; KAWASAKI, M.; GUARRO, J. *Sporothrix brasiliensis*, *S. globosa* and *S. mexicana*, three new *Sporothrix* species of clinical interest. **Journal of Clinical Microbiology**, Washigton, United States, v. 45, n. 10, p. 3198-3206, October, 2007.

MARIMON, R.; GENÉ, J.; CANO, J.; TRILLES, M.; DOS SANTOS, L.; GUARRO, J. Molecular phylogeny of *Sporothrix schenckii*. **Journal of Clinical Microbiology**, Washington, United States, v. 44, n. 9, p.3251-3256, September, 2006.

MARIO, D. N.; GUARRO, J.; SANTURIO, J. M. ALVES, S. H.; CAPILLA, J. *In vitro* and *in vivo* efficacy of amphotericin B combined with posaconazole against experimental disseminated sporotrichosis. **Antimicrobial Agents and Chemotherapy**, Washington, United States, v. 59, n. 8, p. 5018-5021, August, 2015.

MARQUEZ, Beatriz Padrón. **Chemical Components with Bactericidal, Fungicidal and Cytotoxic Activity from Plants of the Myrtaceae and Lauraceae Families**. 86 f. Tesis (Doctorate) - Faculty of Biological Sciences - Universidad Autónoma de Nuevo León, Nuevo León, Mexico, 2010.

MARTiNEZ, M.G.; MARTiNEZ, C.M.; UTRILLA, G.B.; MARTiNEZ, M.N.F. An analysis of the use of liposomal amphotericin B. **Revista Iberoamericina de Micologia**, Barcelona, Spain, v.31, n.2, p.109-113, April/June, 2014.

MARTINS, Anelise Afonso. **Experimental systemic sporotrichosis: *in vivo* evaluation of β -(1-3) glucan and in association with itraconazole in murine model**. Thesis (PhD) - Faculty of Veterinary Medicine, Federal University of Rio Grande do Sul, Porto Alegre/RS, 2012.

MARTIUS, C., EICHLER, A.G., URBAN, I. **Flora Brasiliensis - volume 6(3): fasicle 87** (1882). Available at: http://plantillustrations.org/illustration.php2id_illustration=33474. Accessed on April 5, 2017.

MASCLEF, Amédée. **Atlas des plantes de France : utiles, nuisibles et ornementales : complément**. 4th ed. Belin, Paris, France, 1987.

MASEVHE, N.A.; AWOUAFACK, M.D.; AHMED, A.S.; MCGAW, L.J.; ELOFF, J.N. Clerodendrumic acid, a new triterpenoid from *Clerodendrum glabrum* (Verbenaceae) and antimicrobial activities of fractions and constituents. **Helvetica Chimica Acta**, Basel, Switzerland, v. 96, n. 9, p. 1693-1703, September, 2013.

MASOKO, P.; PICARD, J.; ELOFF, J.N. Antifungal activities of six South African *Terminalia* species (Combretaceae). **Journal of Ethnopharmacology**, Lausanne, Ireland, v. 99, n. 2, p.301-308, June, 2005.

MASOKO, P.; PICARD, J.; ELOFF, J.N. The antifungal activity of twenty-four Southern African *Combretum* species (Combretaceae). **South African Journal of Botany**, Pretoria, South Africa, v.73, n.2, p.173-183, April, 2007.

MASOKO, P.; PICARD, J.; ELOFF, J.N. The use of a rat model to evaluate the *in vivo* toxicity and wound healing activity of selected *Combretum* and *Terminalia* (Combretaceae) species extracts. **The Onderstepoort Journal of Veterinary Research**, Pretoria, South Africa, v. 77, n. 1, p. 1-7, October, 2010.

MASOKO, P.; PICARD, J.; HOWARD, R.L.; MAPURU, L.J.; ELOFF, J.N. *In vivo* antifungal effect of *Combretum* and *Terminalia* species extracts on cutaneous wound healing in immunosuppressed rats. **Pharmaceutical Biology**, London, England, v.48, n.6, p.621-632, June, 2010.

MAWBY, D.I.; WHITTEMORE, J.C.; GENGER, S.; PAPICH, M.G. Bioequivalence of orally administered generic, compounded, and innovator-formulated itraconazole in healthy dogs. **Journal of Veterinary Internal**

Medicine, Philadelphia, United States, v.28, n. 1, p.72-77, January/February, 2014.

MBAKWEM-ANIEBO, C.; ONIANWA, O.; OKONKO, I.O. Effects of *Ocimum gratissimum* leaves on common dermatophytes and causative agent of Pityriasis versicolor in Rivers State, Nigeria. **Journal of Microbiology Research**, Rosemead, United States, v.2, n.4, p. 108-113, 2012.

MCGAW, L.J.; RABE, T.; SPARG, S.G.; JAGER, A.K.; ELOFF, J.N.; VAN STADEN, J. An investigation on the biological activity of *Combretum* species.

Journal of Ethnopharmacology, Lausanne, Ireland, v.75, n.1, p. 45-50, April, 2001.

McGINNIS, M.R.N.; NORDOFF, N.; LI, R.K.; PASARELL, L.; WARNOCK, D.W. *Sporothrix schenckii* sensitivity to voriconazole, itraconazole, and amphotericin B. **Medical Mycology**, Oxford, England, v.39, n 4, p.369-371, August, 2001.

MEINERZ, A. R. M.; NASCENTE, P. S.; SCHUCH, L.F.D.; FARIA, R.O.; SANTIN, R.; CLEFF, M. B.; MADRID, I. M.; MARTINS, A. A.; NOBRE, M. O.; MEIRELES, M. C. A.; MELLO, J. R. B.. Feline sporotrichosis - case report. **Ciência Animal Brasileira**, v. 8, n. 3, p.575-577, July/September, 2007.

MEINERZ, A.R.M.; NASCENTE, P.S.; SCHUCH, L.F.D.; CLEFF, M.B.; SANTIN, R.; BRUM, C. S.; NOBRE, M. O.; MEIRELES, M. C.A.; MELLO, J. R. B. *In vitro* susceptibility of *Sporothrix schenckii* isolates to terbinafine and itraconazole. **Revista da Sociedade Brasileira de Medicina Tropical**, Uberaba, v.40, n.1, p.60-62, January/February, 2007.

MEIRELES, Màrio Carlos Araùjo; NASCENTE, Patricia da Silva. **Veterinary Mycology**. Pelotas: Editora Universitària UFPel, 2009.

MONTENEGRO, H.; RODRIGUES, A.M.; DIAS, M.A.G.; DA SILVA, E.A.; BERNARDI, F.; DE CAMARGO, Z.P. Feline sporotrichosis due to *Sporothrix brasiliensis*: an emerging animal infection in Sâo Paulo, Brazil. **BMC**

Veterinary Research, London, England, v.10, n.269, p.1-11, November, 2014.

MOTSEI, M.L.; LINDSEY, K.L.; VON STADEN, J.; JAGER, A.K. Screening of traditionally used South African plants for antifungal activity against *Candida albicans*. **Journal of Ethnopharmacology**, Lausanne, Ireland, v. 86, n.2-3, p. 235-241, June, 2003.

MOUREY, A.; CANILLAC, N. Anti-Listeria *monocytogenes* activity of essential oils components of conifers. **Food Control**, Kidlington, England, v. 13, n. 4-5, p. 289-292, June/July, 2002.

NARDONI, S.; MUGNAINI, L.; PISTELLI, L.; LEONARDI, M.; SANNA, V.; PERRUCCI, S.; PISSERI, F.; MANCIANTI, F. Clinical and mycological evaluation of an herbal antifungal formulation in canine *Malassezia* dermatitis. **Journal de Mycologie Médicale**, Paris, France, v. 24, n. 3, p. 234-240, September, 2014.

NIKOLIC, M.; JOVANOVIC, K.K.; MARKOVIC, T.; MARKOVIC, D.; GLIGORIJEVIC, N.; RADULOVIC, S.; SOKOVIC, M. Chemical composition, antimicrobial, and cytotoxic properties of five Lamiaceae essential oils. **Industrial Crops and Products**, Amsterdam, Netherlands, v.61, n.1, p.225232, November, 2014.

NOBRE, M. O.; CASTRO, A. P.; CAETANO, D.; SOUZA, L. L.; MEIRELES, M. C. A.; FERREIRO, L.. Recurrence of sporotrichosis in cats with zoonotic involvement. **Revista Iberoamericana de Micologia**, Barcelona, Spain, v. 18, n. 3, p. 137-140, September, 2001.

NOVAK, J., LANGBEHN, J., PANK, F., & FRANZ, C. M. Essential oil compounds in a historical sample of marjoram (*Origanum majorana* L., Lamiaceae). **Flavor and Fragrance Journal**, Firmenich, Switzerland, v. 17, n. 3, p.175-180, May/June, 2002.

ODDS, F.C.; BROWN, A.J.P.; GOW, N.A.R. Antifungal agents: mechanisms of action. **Trends in Microbiology**, Cambridge, England, v.11, n.6, p.272-279, June, 2003.

OJEDA, T.; RODRiGUEZ-PICHARDO, A.; SUAREZ, A.I.; CAMACHO, F.M. Sporotrichosis in Seville (Spain). **Infectious Diseases and Microbiologia Clinica**, Barcelona, Spain, v. 29, n. 3, p. 233-234, March, 2011.

OLADELE, A.T.; DAIRO, B.A.; ELUJOBA, A.A.; OYELAMI, A. Management of superficial fungal infections with *Senna alata* ("alata") soap: a preliminary report. **African Journal of Pharmacy and Pharmacology**, South Africa, v.4, n.3, p.98-103, March, 2010.

OLIVEIRA, D. C.; LORETO, E. S.; MARIO, D. A. N.; LOPES, P. G. M.; NEVES, L. V.; ROCHA, M. P.; SANTURIO, J. M.; ALVES, S. H. *Sporothrix schenckii* complex: susceptibilities to combined antifungal agents and characterization of enzymatic profiles. **Revista do Instituto de Medicina Tropical**, Sao Paulo, v. 57, n. 4, p.289-294,July/August, 2015.

OLIVEIRA, D.C.; LOPES, P.G.; SPADER, T.B.; MAHL, C.D.; TRONCO-ALVES, G.R.; SANTURIO, J.M.; ALVES, S.H. Antifungal Susceptibilities of *Sporothrix albicans*, *S. brasiliensis*, and S. luriei of the *S. schenckii* Complex Identified in Brazil. **Journal of Clinical Microbiology**, Washington, United States, v.49, n.8, p.3047-3049, August, 2011.

OMER, E.A.; HENDAWY, S.F.; EL-DEEN, A.M.N.; ZAKI, F.N.; ABD-ELGAWAD, M.M.; KANDEEL, A.M.; IBRAHIM, A.K.; ISMAIL, R.F. Some biological activities of *Tagetes lucida* plant cultivated in Egypt. **Advances in Environmental Biology**, Punjab, Pakistan, v.9, n.2, p.82-88, January, 2015.

OTSUKA, M.; CASTRO, R.C.C.; MICHALANY, N.S.; LUCAS, R.; LARSSON, C.E.Jr.; LARSSON, C.E. Sporotrichosis in Sao Paulo (Brazil): clinical and epidemiological features. **Veterinary Dermatology**, Oxford, England, v.15, n. 1, p.46, August, 2004.

PELL, Susan Katherine. **Molecular systematics of the cashew family**

(Anacardiaceae). XX f. Thesis (Doctorate) - Louisiana State University, University of Agricultural and Mechanical College, USA, 2004.

PEREIRA, A. S.; SCHUBACH, T. M. P.; GREMIÂO, I. D. F.; SILVA, D. T.; FIGUEIREDO, F. B.; ASSIS, N. V.; PASSOS, S. R. L.. Therapeutic aspects of feline sporotrichosis. **Acta Scientiae Veterinariae**, Porto Alegre, v. 37, n. 4, p. 311-321, 2009.

PEREIRA, S. A.; SILVA, J. N.; GREMIÂO, I. D. F.; FIGUEREDO, F. B.; DUTRA, V. M.; NASCIMENTO, K. C. S.; MATTOS, A. S.; HOLZ, K.; SCHUBACH, T. M. P. Therapeutic response of cats with sporotrichosis treated at the IPEC/FIOCRUZ zoonoses service between 2002 and 2004. **Acta Scientiae Veterinariae**, Porto Alegre, v. 35, n. 2, p. 680-682, 2007.

PIEROZAN, M.K.; PAULETTI, G.F.; ROTA, L.; SANTOS, A.C.A.; LERIN, L.A.; DI LUCCIO, M.; MOSSI, A.J.; ATTI-SERAFINI, L.; CANSIAN, R.L.; OLIVEIRA, J.V. Chemical characterization and antimicrobial activity of essential oils of *Salvia* L. species. **Food Science and Technology**, Campinas, v.29, n.4, p.764-770, December, 2009.

POHLIT, A.M.; PINTO, A.C.S.; MAUSE, R. Pluripotente plant and important phytochemical substance source. **Revista Fitos**, Rio de Janeiro, v. 2, n. 1, p.7-18, June/September, 2006.

PRINS, C.L.; LEMOS, C.L.S.; FREITAS, S.P. Effect of extraction time on the composition and yield of rosemary (*Rosmarinus officinalis*) essential oil. **Revista Brasileira de Plantas Medicinais**, Botucatu, v.8, n. 4, p.92-95, December, 2006.

RAMiREZ SOTO, M.C. Sporotrichosis: The Story of an Endemic Region in Peru over 28 Years (1985 to 2012). **PLoS One**, San Francisco, United States, v. 10, n. 6, p.e0127924, June, 2015.

RAMOS-E-SILVA, M.; VASCONCELOS, C.; CARNEIRO, S.; CESTARI, T. Sporothricosis. **Clinics in Dermatology**, Philadelphia, United States, v. 25, n.

2, p.181-187, March/April, 2007.

REES, R.K.; SWARTZBERG, J.E. Feline-transmitted sporotrichosis: A case study from California. **Dermatology Online Journal**, Davis, United States, v. 17, n. 6, p. 2, June, 2011.

REIS, E. G.; GREMIÃO, I. D. F.; KITADA, A. A. B.; ROCHA, R. F. D. B.; CASTRO, V. S. P.; BARROS, M. B. L.; MENEZES, R. C.; PEREIRA, S. A.; SCHUBACH, T. M. P. Potassium iodide capsule treatment of feline sporotrichosis. **Journal of Feline Medicine and Surgery**, London, England, v. 14, n. 6, p. 399-404, June, 2012.

RIVIERE, Jim E.; PAPICH, Mark G. **Veterinary Pharmacology and Therapeutics**. 9th ed. Ioza State University Press: Ames, USA, 2009.

RODRIGUES, A.M.; CHOAPPA, R.C.; FERNANDES, G.F.; DE HOOG, G.S.; DE CAMARGO, Z.P. *Sporothrix chilensis* sp. nov. (Ascomycota: Ophiostomatales), a soil-borne agent of human sporotrichosis with mild-pathogenic potential to mammals. **Fungal Biology**, Amsterdam, Netherlands, v. 120, n. 2, p.246-264, February, 2016.

RODRIGUES, A.M.; DE HOOG, G.; ZHANG, Y.; CAMARGO, Z.P. Emerging sporotrichosis in driven by clonal and recombinant *Sporothrix* species. **Emerging Microbes and Infections**, New York, United States, v.3, n.5, p. e32, May, 2014.

RODRIGUES, A.M.; DE MELO, T.M.; DE HOOG, G.S.; SCHUBACH, T.M.P.; PEREIRA, S.A.; FERNANDES, G.F.; BEZERRA, L.M.L.; FELIPE, M.S.; CAMARGO, Z.P. Phylogenetic analysis reveals a high prevalence of *Sporothrix brasiliensis* in feline sporotrichosis outbreaks. **PLoS Neglected Tropical Diseases**, San Francisco, United States, v. 7, n. 6, p. e2281, June, 2013.

ROJAS, R.; BUSTAMANTE, B.; BAUER, J.; FERNANDEZ, I.; ALBAN, J.; LOCK, O. Antimicrobial activity of selected Peruvian medicinal plants. **Journal**

of Ethnopharmacology, London, England, v.88, n. 2-3, p.199-204, October, 2003.

ROSSI, C.N.; ODAGUIRI, J.; LARSSON, C.E. Retrospective assessment of the treatment of sporotrichosis in cats and dogs using itraconazole. **Acta Scientiae Veterinariae**, Porto Alegre, n. 42, p.1114, 2013.

RUTTER, Richard .A. **Catàlogo de Plantas Utiles de la Amazonia Peruana**. ILV: Lima, Peru, 1990.

SAIKIA, D.; KHANUJA, S.P.S.; KAHOL, A.P.; GUPTA, S.C.; KUMAR, S. Comparative antifungal activity of essential oils and constituents from three distinct genotypes of *Cymbopogon* spp. **Current Science**, Bangalore, India, v.80, n.10, p.1264-1266, May, 2001.

SANCHEZ, Ana Margarita Garcia. **Inhibition of *Sporothrix schenckii* by legume species popularly used in Guatemala for the treatment of mycosis**. Guatemala City. 54 f. Thesis (Doctorate) - Faculty of Chemical Sciences and Pharmacy, University of San Carlos de Guatemala, 2009.

SANDHU, K.; GUPTA, S.; Potassium iodide remains the most effective therapy for cutaneous sporotrichosis. **Journal of Dermatological Treatment**, Houndmills, England, v. 14, n. 4, p. 200-202, December, 2003.

SANTANA, D.B.; COSTA, R.C.; ARAÙJO, R.M.; PAULA, J.E.; SILVEIRA, E.R.; BRAZ-FILHO, R.; ESPINDOLA, L. S. Activity of Fabaceae species extracts against fungi and Leishmania: vatacarpan as a novel potent anti- *Candida* agent. **Revista Brasileira de Farmacognosia**, Sâo Paulo, v.25, n.4, p. 401-406, July/August, 2015.

SARAC, N.; UGUR, A. The *in vitro* antimicrobial activities of the essential oils of some Lamiaceae species from Turkey. **Journal of Medicinal Food**, Larchmont, United States, v.12, n.4, p.902-907, September, 2009.

SCHUBACH, A.; BARROS, M.B.; WANKE, B. Epidemic sporotrichosis. **Current Opinion in Infectious Diseases**, Hagerstown, United States, v. 21,

n. 2, p.129-133, April, 2008.

SCHUBACH, T. M. P.; MENEZES, R. C.; WANKE, B. **Sporotrichosis**. In: Greene C.E. (Ed). Infectious diseases of the dog and cat. 4th edition. Philadelphia: W.B. Saunders Company, p.645-650, 2012.

SCHUBACH, T.M.P.; SCHUBACH, A.; OKAMOTO, T.; BARROS, M.B.; FIGUEIREDO, F.B.; CUZZI, T.; FIALHO-MONTEIRO, P.C.; REIS, R.S., PEREZ, M.A.; WANKE, B. Evaluation of an epidemic of sporotrichosis in cats: 347 cases (1998-2001). **Journal of the American Veterinary Medical Association**, Ithaca, United States, v.224, n.10, p.1623-1629. May, 2004.

SCOTT, D.; MILLER, W.; GRIFFIN, C. **Muller and Kirk's Small Animal Dermatology**. 6th edition. Phyladelphia: W. B. Saunders, 2001.

SCOTT, D.W.; MILLER, W.H.; GRIFFIN, C. **Dermatologia de Pequenos Animais**, Rio de Janeiro: Interlivros,1996.

SERAFINI, L. A. et al. **Extractions and applications of essential oils from aromatic and medicinal plants.** Caxias do Sul: EDUCS, 2002

SHAI, L.J.; McGAW, L.J.; ADEROGBA, M.A.; MDEE, L.K.; ELOFF, J.N. Four pentacyclic triterpenoids with antifungal and antibacterial activity from *Curtisia dentata* (Burm.f) C.A. Sm. leaves. **Journal of Ethnopharmacology**, Lausanne, Ireland, v.119, n. 2, p.238-244, September, 2008.

SHARMA, N. L.; MEHTA, K. I. S.; MAHAJAN, V. K.; KANGA, A. K.; SHARMA, V. C.; TEGTA G. R.. Cutaneous sporotrichosis of face: polymorphism and reactivation after intralesional triamcinolone. **Indian Journal of Dermatology, Venereology and Leprology**, Mumbai, India, v. 73, n. 3, p. 188-190, 2007.

SILVA, D. T.; PEREIRA, S. A.; GREMIÂO, I. D. F.; CHAVES, A. R.; CAVALCANTI, M. C. H.; SILVA, J. N.; SCHUBACH, T. M. P. Sporotrichosis feline conjunctival. **Acta Scientae Veterinariae**, Porto Alegre, v. 36, n. 2, p. 181-184, 2008.

SILVA, D.T.; MENEZES, R.C.; GREMIÂO, I.D.F.; SCHUBACH, T.M.P.;

BOECHAT, J.S.; PEREIRA, A.S. Zoonotic sporotrichosis: biosafety procedures. **Acta Scientiae Veterinariae**, Porto Alegre, v.40, n.4, p.1067, 2012.

SILVA, J.P.; SIQUEIRA, A.M. Accion antibacteriana de extratos hidroalcohólicos de *Rubus urticaefolius*. **Revista Cubana de Plantas Medicinais**, Ciudad de la Habana, v. 5, n. 1, p.26-29, January/April, 2000.

SILVA, Margarete Bernardo Tavares da. **Socio-spatial distribution of human sporotrichosis in patients treated at the Evandro Chagas Clinical Research Institute between 1997 and 2007, living in the state of Rio de Janeiro**. 143 f. Dissertation (Master's Degree) - Public Health Sciences, Oswaldo Cruz Foundation, Rio de Janeiro/RJ, 2010.

SILVA, O., DUARTE, A., CABRITA, J., PIMENTEL, M., DINIZ, A., GOMES, E. Antimicrobial activity of Guinea-Bissau traditional remedies. **Journal of Ethnopharmacology**, Lausanne, Ireland, v. 50, n. 1, p. 55-59, January, 1996.

SIMOES, Claudia M. Oliveira et al. **Pharmacognosy: from the plant to the medicine**. 5.ed. Porto Alegre: Editora da UFRGS, 2003.

SINHA, G.K.; GULATI, B.C. Antibacterial and antifungal study of some essential oils and some of their constituents. **Indian Perfumer**, Kanpur, India, v.34, n.2, p.126-129, November, 1990.

SMITH, J.A.; PAPICH, M.G.; RUSSELL, G.; MITCHELL, M.A. Effects of compounding on pharmacokinetics of itraconazole in black-footed penguins (*Spheniscus demersus*). **Journal of Zoo and Wildlife Medicine**, Lawrence, United States, v.41, n.3, p.487-495, September, 2010.

SOARES, I.H.; LORETO, É.S.; ROSSATO, L.; MARIO, D.N.; VENTURINI, T.P.; BALDISSERA, F.; SANTURIO, J.M.; ALVES, S.H. *In vitro* activity of essential oils extracted from condiments against fluconazole-resistant and -sensitive *Candida glabrata*. **Journal de Mycologie Médicale**, Paris, France, v. 25, n. 3, p. 213-217, September, 2015.

SOUZA, C. P.; LUCAS, R.; RAMADINHA, R. H. R.; PIRES, T. B. C. P. Cryosurgery in association with itraconazole for the treatment of feline sporotrichosis. **Journal of Feline Medicine and Surgery**, London, England, v. 18, n. 2, p.137-143, February, 2016.

SOUZA, E. L.; STAMFORD, T. L. M.; LIMA, E. O.; TRAJANO, V. N. Effectiveness of *Origanum vulgare* L. essential oil to inhibit the growth of food spoiling yeasts. **Food Control**, Kidlington, England, v. 18, p.409-413, May, 2007.

SOUZA, N. T.; NASCIMENTO, A. C. B. M.; SOUZA, J. O, T,; SANTOS, F. C. G. C.A.; CASTRO, R. B.. Canine sporotrichosis: case report. **Arquivo Brasileiro de Medicina Veterinària e Zootecnia**, Belo Horizonte, v. 61, n. 3, p. 572-576, June, 2009.

SPINOSA, Helenice de Souza et al. **Farmacologia Aplicada à Medicina Veterinària**. 4 ed. Rio de Janeiro: Guanabara Koogan, 2006.

STEIN, A.C.; ALVAREZ, S.; AVANCINI, C.; ZACCHINO, C.; VON POSER, G. Antifungal activity of some coumarins obtained from species of *Pterocaulon* (Asteraceae). **Journal of Ethnopharmacology**, Lausanne, Ireland, v. 107, n. 1, p. 95-98, August, 2006.

STEIN, A.C.; SORTINO, M.; AVANCINI, C.; ZACCHINO, S.; VON POSER, G. Ethnoveterinary medicine in the search for antimicrobial agents: antifungal activity of some species of *Pterocaulon* (Asteraceae). **Journal of Ethnopharmacology**, Lausanne, Ireland, v. 99, n. 2, p. 211-214, June, 2005.

STOPIGLIA, C. D. O.; MAGAGNIN, C. M.; CASTRILLÓN, M. R.; MENDES, S. D. C., HEIDRICH, D.; VALENTE, P.; SCROFERNEKER, M. L.. Antifungal susceptibilities and identification of species of the *Sporothrix schenckii* complex isolated in Brazil. **Medical Mycology**, Oxford, England, v. 52, n. 1, p. 56-64, January, 2014.

STOPIGLIA, C.D.O.; VIANNA, D.R.; MEIRELLES, G.C.; TEIXEIRA, H.; VON

POSER, G.L.; SCROFERNEKER, M.L. Antifungal activity of *Pterocaulon* species (Asteraceae) against *Sporothrix schenckii*. **Journal de Mycologie Médicale**, Paris, France, v.21, n. 3, p.169-172, September, 2011.

SULEIMAN, M.M.; McGAW, L.J.; NAIDOO, V.; ELOFF, J.N. Evaluation of several tree species for activity against the animal fungal pathogen *Aspergillus fumigatus*. **South African Journal of Botany**, Pretoria, South Africa, v.76, n.1, p.64-71, January, 2009.

SULEIMAN, M.M.; NAIDOO, V.; ELOFF, J.N. Preliminary screening of some fractions of *Loxostylis alata* (Anacardiaceae) for antimicrobial and antioxidant activities. **African Journal of Biotechnology**, Lagos, Nigeria, v. 11, n. 9, p. 2340-2348, January, 2012.

TEPE, B.; DONNEY, E.; UNLU, M.; CANDAN, F.; DAFERERA, D.; UNLU, GV.; POLISSIOU, M.; SOKMEN, A. Antimicrobial and antioxidative activities of the essential oils and methanol extracts of *S. cryptantha* (Montbret et Aucher ex Benth.) *S. multicaulis* (Vahl.). **Food Chemistry**, Berlin, Germany, v. 84, n. 4, p. 519-525, 2004.

TILLEY, L. P.; SMITH, F. W. K. Jr. **Veterinary consultation in 5 minutes Canine and feline species**, 2nd edition. Barueri: Manole, 2003.

TOPÇU, G. Bioactive triterpenoids from *Salvia* species. **Journal of Natural Products**, Cincinnati, United States, v. 69, n. 3, p.482-487, March, 2006.

TREW, C.J.; EHRET, G.D. **Plantae Selectae - volume 5** (1755). Available at: http://plantillustrations.org/illustration.php?id_illustration=58541. Accessed on: 05 April 2017.

TRILLES, L.; FÉRNANDEZ-TORRES, B.; DOS SANTOS LAZERA, M.; WANKE, B.; SCHUBACH, A. O.; PAES, R. A.; INZA, I.; GUARRO, J. *In vitro* antifungal susceptibilities of *Sporothrix schenckii* in two growth phases. **Antimicrobial Agents and Chemotherapy**, Washington, United States, v. 49, n. 9, p. 3952-3954, September, 2005.

UNLU, M.; VANDAR-UNLU, G.; VURAL, N.; DONMEZ, E.; OZBAS, Z.Y. Chemical composition, antibacterial and antifungal activity of the essential oil of *Thymbra spicata* L. from Turkey. **Natural Products Research**, Milton Park, England, v.23, n.6, p.572-579, 2009.

VALENTE, J.; ZUZARTE, M.; GONÇALVES, M.J.; LOPES, M.C.; CAVALEIRO, C.; SALGUEIRO, L.; CRUZ, M.T. Antifungal, antioxidant and anti-inflammatory activities of *Oenanthe crocata* L. essential oil. **Food and Chemical Toxicology**, Oxford, England, v.62, p.349-352, December, 2013.

VAN WYK, Bem-Erik; VAN OUDTSHOORN, Bosch; GERICKE, Nigel. **Medicinal Plants of South Africa**. 2th ed. Briza Publications: Pretoria, South Africa, 2012.

VENKATESAN, M.; VISWANATHAN, M.B.; RAMESH, N.; LAKSHMANAPERUMALSAMY, P. Antibacterial potential from Indian *Suregada angustifolia*. **Journal of Ethnopharmacology**, Lausanne, Ireland, v. 99, n. 3, p. 349-352, July, 2005.

VERASTEGUI, A.; VERDE, J.; GARCIA, S.; HEREDIA, N.; ORANDAY, A.; RIVAS, C. Species of *Agave* with antimicrobial activity against selected pathogenic bacteria and fungi. **World Journal of Microbiology and Biotechnology**, Berlin, Germany, v.24, n. 7, p.1249-1252, July, 2008.

VERASTEGUI, M.A.; SANCHEZ, C.A.; HEREDIA, N.L.; GARCIA- ALVARADO, J.S. Antimicrobial activity of extracts of three major plants from the Chihuahuan desert. **Journal of Ethnopharmacology**, Lausanne, ireland, v.52, n.3, p.175-177, July, 1996.

VERMA, S.; VERMA, G.K.; SiNGH, G.; KANGA, A.; SHANKER, V.; SiNGH, D.; GUPTA, P.; MOKTA, K.; SHARMA, V. Sporotrichosis in sub-himalayan india. **PLoS Neglected Tropical Diseases**, San Francisco, United States, v. 6, n.6, e1673, June, 2012.

VIETZ, F.B. **Icones Plantarum Medico-Oeconomico-Technologicarum -**

volume 2 (1804) Available at: http://plantillustrations.org/illustration.php2id illustration=152309. Accessed on: April 05, 2017.

VUKOViC, N.; SUKDOLAK, S.; SOLUJUC, S.; NiCiFOROViC, N. Antimicrobial activity of the essential oil obtained from roots and chemical composition of the volatile constituents from the roots, stems, and leaves of *Ballota nigra* from Serbia. **Journal of Medicinal Food**, Larchmont, United States, v. 12, n. 2, p. 435-441, April, 2009.

WATANABE, M.; HAYAMA, K.; FUJiTA, H.; YAGOSHi, M.; YARiTA, K.; KAMEi, K.; TERUi, T. A case of sporotrichosis caused by *Sporothrix globosa* in Japan. **Annals of Dermatology**, Seoul, Korea, v. 28, n.2, p. 251-252, April, 2016.

WALLER, S.B.; PETER, C.M.; HOFFMANN, J.F.; PICOLI, T.; OSÓRIO, L.D.; CHAVES, F.; ZANI, J.L.; DE FARIA, R.O.; DE MELLO, J.R.; MEIRELES, M.C. Chemical and cytotoxic analyses of brown Brazilian propolis (*Apis mellifera*) and its *in vitro* activity against itraconazole-resistant *Sporothrix brasiliensis*. **Microbial Pathogenesis**, London, England, v. 105, p. 117-121, April, 2017.

WALLER, S.B.; MADRID, I.M.; CLEFF, M.B.; SANTIN, R.; FREITAG, R.A.; MEIRELES, M.C.A.; MELLO, J.R.B. Effects of essential oils of *Rosmarinus officinalis* Linn. and *Origanum vulgare* Linn. from different origins on *Sporothrix brasiliensis* and *Sporothrix schenckii* complex. **Arquivo Brasileiro de Medicina Veterinària e Zootecnia**, Belo Horizonte, v. 68, n. 4, p. 991999, July/August, 2016.

WALLER, S.B.; MADRID, I.M.; FERRAZ, V.; PICOLI, T.; CLEFF, M.B.; FARIA, R.O.; MEIRELES, M.C.A.; MELLO, J.R.B. Cytotoxicity and anti- *Sporothrix brasiliensis* activity of the *Origanum majorana* Linn. oil. **Brazilian Journal of Microbiology**, Sao Paulo, v. 47, n. 4, p. 896-901, October/December, 2016.

WALLER, S.B.; MADRID, I.M.; SERRA, E.F.; GOMES, A.R.; CLEFF, M.B.;

FARIA, R.O. *In vitro* susceptibility of the *Sporothrix brasiliensis* to aqueous extracts of green-tea (*Camellia sinensis* L. Kuntze). **Acta Veterinaria Brasilica**, Mossoró, v. 9, n. 4, p. 342-347, December, 2015.

WEINGART, C.; LÜBKE-BECKER, A.; KOHN, B. *Sporothrix schenckii* infection in a cat. **Berliner und Münchener tierarztliche Wochenschrift**, Berlin, Germany, v. 123, n. 3-4, p. 125-129, March/April, 2010.

WEN, L.; HADDAD, M.; FERNANDEZ, I.; ESPINOZA, G.; RUIZ, C.; NEYRA, E.; BUSTAMANTE, B.; ROJAS, R. Antifungal activity of four plants used in traditional Peruvian medicine. Analysis of 3'-Formyl-2'4'6'-Trihydroxyhydrochalcone, the active principle of *Psidium acutangulum*. **Revista de la Sociedad Quimica del Perù**, Lima, Peru, v.77, n.3, p.199-204, 2011.

WERNER, A. H.; WERNER, B. E.. Sporotrichosis in man and animal. **International Journal of Dermatology**, Oxford, England, v. 33, n. 10, p. 692-700, October, 1994.

WHITTEMORE, J. C.; WEBB, C. B. Successful treatment of nasal sporotrichosis in a dog. **The Canadian Veterinary Journal**, Ottawa, Canada, v. 48, n. 4, p. 411-414, April, 2007.

WOJCIECHOWSKI, M.F.; LAVIN, M.; SANDESRSON, M.J. A phylogeny of Legumes (Leguminosae) based on analysis of the plastid MATK gene resolves many well-supported subclades within the family. **American Journal of Botany**, Baltimore, United States, v. 91, n. 11, p. 1846-1862, November, 2004.

WOOD, J.M.; EVANS, M.S. **Natal Plants - volume 4** (1903-1906).

Available at:

http://plantillustrations.org/illustration.php2id illustration=192226. Accessed on: April 05, 2017.

WOODVILLE, W.; HOOKER, W.J.; SPRATT, G. **Medical Botany - volume 3** (1832). Available at:< http://plantillustrations.org/illustration.php2id

illustration=81262. Accessed on: 05 April 2017.

XAVIER, M.O.; NOBRE, M.O.; SAMPAIO JR. ANTUNES, T. A.; NASCENTE, P. D. S.; SÓRIA, F. B. D. A.; MEIRELES, M. C. A.. Feline sporotrichosis with human involvement in the city of Pelotas, RS, Brazil. **Ciência Rural**, Santa Maria, v. 34, n. 6, p. 1961-1963, November/December, 2004.

YEGNESWARAN, P.P.; SRIPATHI, H.; BAIRY, I., LONIKAR, V.; RAO, R.; PRABHU, S. Zoonotic sporotrichosis of lymphocutaneous type in a man acquired from a domesticated feline source: report of a first case in southern Karnataka, India. **International Journal of Dermatology**, Oxford, England, v. 48, n. 11, p. 1198-1200. November, 2009.

ZAIDI, M.A.; CROW JR., S.A. Biologically active traditional medicinal herbs from Balochistan, Pakistan. **Journal of Ethnopharmacology**, Lausanne, Ireland, v. 96, n. 1-2, p. 331-334, January, 2005.

ZHANG, X.; HUANG, H.; FENG, P.; ZHANG, J.; ZHONG, Y.; XUE, R.; XIE, Z; LI, M.; XI, L. *In vitro* activity of itraconazole in combination with terbinafine against clinical strains of itraconazole-insensitive *Sporothrix schenckii*. **European Journal of Dermatology**, Montrouge, France, v. 21, n. 4, p. 573576, July/August, 2011.

ZIELINSKA, S.; MATKOWSKI, A. Phytochemistry and bioactivity of aromatic and medicinal plants from the genus *Agastache* (Lamiaceae). **Phytochemistry Reviews**, Dordrecht , Netherlands, v. 13, n. 2, p. 391-416, June, 2014.

ZUZARTE, M.; GONÇALVES, M.J.; CAVALEIRO, C.; CRUZ, M.T.; BENZARTI, A.; MARONGIU, B.; MAXIA, A. PIRAS, A.; SALGUEIRO, L. Antifungal and anti-inflammatory potential of *Lavandula stoechas* and *Thymus herba-barona* essential oils. **Industrial Crops and Products**, Amsterdam, Netherlands, v. 44, p. 97-103, January, 2013.

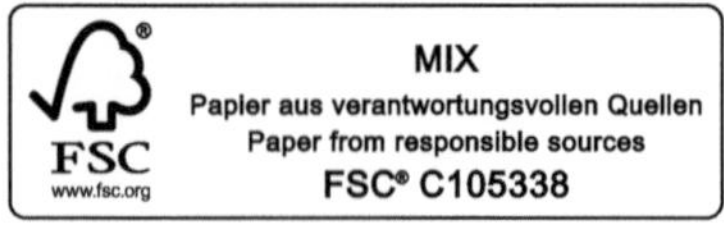

Printed by Books on Demand GmbH, Norderstedt / Germany